Gestalt Practice:
Living and Working
in Pursuit of wHolism

Gestalt Practice:
Living and Working
in Pursuit of wHolism

First published in 2019 by Libri Publishing.

Copyright © Libri Publishing Ltd.

Authors retain the rights to individual chapters.

ISBN 978-1-911450-40-5

All rights reserved. No part of this publication may be reproduced, stored in any retrieval system or transmitted in any form or by any means, electronic, mechanical, photocopying, recording or otherwise, without the prior written permission of the copyright holder for which application should be addressed in the first instance to the publishers. No liability shall be attached to the author, the copyright holder or the publishers for loss or damage of any nature suffered as a result of reliance on the reproduction of any of the contents of this publication or any errors or omissions in its contents.

A CIP catalogue record for this book is available from The British Library

Cover and book design by Carnegie Publishing

Libri Publishing
Brunel House
Volunteer Way
Faringdon
Oxfordshire
SN7 7YR

Tel: +44 (0)845 873 3837

www.libripublishing.co.uk

Contents

DEDICATION	vi
ACKNOWLEDGEMENTS	viii
FOREWORD *Carolyn J. Lukensmeyer*	x
A REFLECTION OF GESTALT PRACTICE: A SHORT VERSION OF MY MISUNDERSTANDING OF GESTALT *Peter Block*	xiv
INTRODUCTION *Mary Ann Rainey and Brenda B. Jones*	xvi

I ROOTS OF GESTALT PRACTICE
 Chapter 1   Edwin C. Nevis Interview – The Cycle of
   Experience   3
 Chapter 2   The Relevance of Gestalt Principles and
   Theory to Organization Development Consultation
   W. Warner Burke   11
 Chapter 3   Gestalt as a Living Spiritual Practice?
   Paul Barber   27

II THE GESTALT PRACTITIONER
 Chapter 4   A Short Note on the "Use-of-Self" and Gestalt
   Mee-Yan Cheung-Judge   41
 Chapter 5   Four Roles of the Gestalt Intervener:
   Holistic Presence Using Experiential Learning Theory
   Mary Ann Rainey   59

III GESTALT PRACTICE AT MULTIPLE LEVELS OF SYSTEM

A. INDIVIDUAL LEVEL OF SYSTEM
 Chapter 6   Navigating the Inner Emotional Landscape in a
   Globalized World *Eva Roettgers*   77
 Chapter 7   Preventing the Tragedy of the Commons:
   A Call to Gestalt OD Practitioners to Pursue Holism for the
   Renewal of our Global Systems *Kate Cowie*   93
 Chapter 8   Gestalt Coaching for Awareness Management:
   The Elements of Mastery *Dorothy E. Siminovitch*   109

Chapter 9   The Executive's Gestalt *Ollie Malone, Jr.*   123

B. WORKING WITH GROUPS
Chapter 10   I'm Better When I Move: Facilitating Movement and Energy in Groups from a Gestalt Perspective *Walt Hopkins*   141

C. LARGE COMPLEX SOCIAL SYSTEMS
Chapter 11   The Cape Cod Model in Organizational Settings *Joseph Melnick*   153
Chapter 12   Gestalt Practice in Large Complex Social Systems: Communities, Clans, Tribes and Other Collective Cultural Configurations *Chantelle Wyley*   167
Chapter 13   Case Study: A Holistic Strategy to Promote Change in a Multinational Corporation *Eugenio Molini*   183

IV GESTALT APPROACH TO CHANGE
Chapter 14   A Gestalt Approach to Optimizing Competence During a Digital Transformation *Gudrun Frank*   197
Chapter 15   Leading Change: A Gestalt Perspective *Jonno Hanafin*   211
Chapter 16   A Systemic Gestalt Supporting Transformational Change Using the Six Cs *Brenda B. Jones*   225
Chapter 17   Gestalt in Organizations: Experiences from Practice in West Africa Cultural Underpinnings of Resistances in Organizational Change: Lessons from Gestalt OD Practice in West Africa *John Nkum and Dan K. B. Inkoom*   241

AFTERWORD *Robert J. Marshak*   249

GESTALT GLOSSARY OF GESTALT THEORY, PRINCIPLES, MODELS AND TERMS   253

INDEX   269

To the memory of Dr. Edwin C. Nevis

(May 20, 1926 – May 20, 2011)

Our teacher and mentor who dedicated his life to taking Gestalt theory and practice to the global masses

Acknowledgements

Mary Ann Rainey

First, I acknowledge my husband Elias Tolbert who has been with me every step of the way. Never once did he say "stop reading," "stop writing," "don't do it." Instead, he kept encouraging me to "finish your book." He knows how to give unconditional love and has taught me how small bits of kindness can be so big. Thank you Honey.

Next to my two sons, Elias Jr. and Jason and the rest of my family for simply believing in me.

Thanks to my editing partner, Brenda B. Jones. I have known Brenda since 1988 when we first met at an NTL new members meeting. We became instant girlfriends. Life threw me some major curves on the way to finishing this book. Brenda did not flinch. She held steady, as she always does, providing comfort and support. Still, we laughed a lot. The moments of giggle were both invigorating and nurturing. I remain in awe of Brenda's knowledge and dedication to the field of applied behavioral science. She loves what she does and sure knows how to do it. I could not have had a better partner.

I owe immense gratitude to Pat Arnold who worked tirelessly on this project. With Pat, it does not matter if it is day or night, when I reach out to her, she responds.

To my colleagues and to my teachers who showed me the way: John D. Carter, Edwin Nevis, Gwen (Sharada) Wade, Claire Stratford, Elaine Kepner, Carolyn j. Lukensmeyer, and Lynne Kweder.

To my dear friend and life-long partner in Gestalt, Jonno Hanafin. Even when we say "enough," we never leave. Also, my gratitude goes to two other partners, John Nkum and Chantelle Wyley, who so eloquently expand my ideas about Gestalt in the world. I always extend a word of gratitude to Dave Kolb for his on-going mentorship.

Thanks to everyone at Libri. The easy manner of Paul Jervis was reassuring as we began our early conversations about this book. Thanks also to Celia Cozens and John Sivak for their patience as we kept pushing deadlines.

And to the colleagues who contributed chapters, thanks for your willingness to take time from your families and busy lives to support this project. We could not have done it without you.

Brenda B. Jones

I would like to thank my Gestalt colleagues and the Gestalt community. I hope this book rises to meet your expectations as our journeys live in our practices and our lifetimes. While working on this book it was my excitement about our intellectual energy, curiosity about the world, being in full contact and having a presence as a community that has been inspiring. My gratitude to you is embedded deeply in my values and practice of Gestalt and OD. I am proud to carry on and to be part of a community that does its own work and wants to make a difference in the world.

Early on as a new student of Gestalt and OD, a number of Gestalt faculty were also NTL faculty members who influenced the course of my work and my life. They are some of the models of good practice that I carry with me to this day. I am profoundly grateful to all of them and, in addition to Edwin Nevis, wish to thank John Carter, Carolyn J. Lukensmeyer and Gwen (Sarada) Gibbs Wade. Although not an NTL member, Claire Stratford represented a special kind of care and devotion to the development of my work.

At Libri Publishers we were fortunate to work with Paul Jervis, Celia Cozens, John Sivak, and the whole team who were behind the scenes. We want to thank our reviewers and endorsers for their commitment to this project and book.

I am grateful to Mary Ann Rainey for being a faithful editing and writing partner over many years and to Patricia Arnold for her work on this project. I am grateful to Mary Blum Rusk who, as a friend and colleague, supports me, and my work, and has for decades.

I am most fortunate in my family life. My husband, Bill, my son Brian, my daughter, Robyn, and their families, make my work life and my career possible. They are generous with their interest in and support of me. Their understanding and loyalty are foundations of the strength I need to successfully serve my clients and make my way in the workplaces of the world. I am comforted by their kindness and care. I know that each day I can be better and do better because they are my family.

We wish to thank Kubeshni Govender for the artistic rendering of the word "wHolism" as used in the title of the book.

Foreword

Carolyn J. Lukensmeyer

I was fortunate to discover Gestalt philosophy, theory and methodology as a very young person. It has informed my approach to making a difference in the world for 50 years and has been an anchor on my lifelong journey to becoming all of who I am. I was particularly pleased and honored to be invited to write the foreword to this significant contribution to the application of Gestalt principles and methods in organizations as I am part of the direct lineage from the originators of Gestalt theory and practice to the fourth and fifth generations of practitioners as represented by the editors, Mary Ann Rainey and Brenda B. Jones and all but one of the authors of chapters in this book.

I was trained at the Gestalt Institute of Cleveland in the early 70s by an esteemed faculty including Erving and Miriam Polster, Sonia and Edwin Nevis, Bill Warner, Cynthia Harris, Marjorie Creelman, and Elaine Kepner; all of whom were trained by Fritz Perls, Laura Perls and Isadore From.

Upon the completion of my training I was honored to become the youngest faculty member of the Gestalt Institute of Cleveland and in that capacity was privileged to be part of an extraordinary cross generational team including Ed Nevis, Elaine Kepner, John Carter, Leonard Hirsch and myself. The five of us spent five days at the Nevis' beautiful home on the ocean on Cape Cod and poured our hearts and minds into the creation of a curriculum that we believed had the potential to move Gestalt beyond its application to individuals into the world of complex systems. That work was one of the most generative collaborations of my career and has, over the ensuing decades, had an impact far beyond what any of us imagined at the time.

Some years later Ed Nevis and I launched the Gestalt International Program in Germany at the invitation of Jurgen Ferchland and Eva Roettgers. I am proud to say that both of these training programs continue to thrive and spread the practice of using Gestalt theory and methodology to transform organizations worldwide.

The editors of this book, Mary Ann Rainey and Brenda B. Jones, have dedicated their careers to expanding the reach of Gestalt theory and practice to all regions of the globe. Their own practices and the work of the people they have trained demonstrate how the roots of Gestalt theory and methodology combined with an understanding of levels of system are powerful tools for effecting change despite the profound cultural differences across the continents.

FOREWORD

Brenda and Mary Ann have intentionally selected authors whose work spans the globe and highlights specific aspects of Gestalt theory and practice applied to organizations. Readers will discover the wisdom of their selections as the range of cases represent so many different contexts and unique perspectives. You are given a window into those aspects of Gestalt theory and methodology that touch some universal truths about what it means to be a human being and how the structures and processes we create in organizations and institutions both limit and expand human experience and our ability to live and work collectively in ways that, as Martin Luther King, Jr. so eloquently expressed, move the moral arc of the universe toward justice.

We are living in a time of great disruption and upheaval. There are serious threats to our way of life, our core institutions and even our very existence at the global level. The stakes are very high whether you are working with individuals and families, groups and organizations, or large complex social or institutional systems. Each of the chapters in this book demonstrates that Gestalt theory and practice can make a significant contribution to the changes that are necessary to deal with dysfunction and achieve a higher level of integration and effectiveness.

For the past 34 years my practice has been dedicated to large-scale change in governance systems in the public sector: first serving as chief of staff to the governor of Ohio – the first woman to hold that position – then serving as part of the transition team and working in the Office of Chief of Staff in the White House of the United States in the early years of the Bill Clinton-Al Gore Administration. In 1995, I gave up my desk in the west wing of the White House in order to found AmericaSpeaks, a nonprofit organization dedicated to bringing citizens back to their rightful position at the table as written in our Declaration of Independence and our Constitution. "We the people" are the foundation of the governance system that created our republic.

While leading AmericaSpeaks and Global Voices for 18 years, working in all 50 states and 33 countries on six continents demonstrating over and over again that when you bring a demographically representative group of people to the table, provide them with factual information representing all ideological perspectives, and when decision makers are committed to participate and listen to the discussion and collective decisions of the people, amazing things can happen. Two profound examples in my home country were "Listening to the City" which brought together 5000 people after the September 11, 2001 (911) terrorist attacks in New York City to make recommendations on the rebuilding of Lower Manhattan; and 3500 people in New Orleans after Katrina and the flooding to determine priorities in the recovery process. In both cases, decision makers embraced the collective decisions of the public. Everything already exists that we need to evolve our political decision-making structures that will give citizens their rightful seat at the table in governance decisions. What is missing is the political will to allow and enable this to happen.

In January 2011, after the tragic mass shooting in Tucson, Arizona, during which six people were killed and 13 others seriously wounded, including former United States Representative Gabrielle Giffords, the community and the University of Arizona quickly came together and created the National Institute for Civil Discourse (NICD) to make something good come out of this horrible tragedy. In July 2012, I was delighted to be selected as the first Executive Director of NICD.

Over the last six and half years, it has been an honor to lead and build the Institute into a force for good in the degraded state of US politics. At NICD we work with elected officials at both the state and national levels, we work with journalists and the media and we work with the American public. It is from this position of influence that I would like to share some of our experience of the power of Gestalt principles and methods as applied in the Institute's work.

Gestalt theory is deeply grounded in wholism and the understanding that for authentic change that can be sustained over time, there are three equally important elements that must be worked with: the organism, in this case the organization/institution; it's environment/context; and the boundary between them. All are equally important to developing interventions that lead to positive change.

Let me take just one basic Gestalt principle and share the power it can bring to working in complex public sector organizations and institutions. That principle is "figure/ground."

Whether it is in the halls of the US Congress or around many multi-generational family dinner tables at Thanksgiving; when the frame of reference is politics, what people see as "figure" when they encounter each other is Republican or Democrat, conservative or liberal, for or against the wall or climate change or any other important public policy issue which has two, dug-in opposing sides. And in far too many instances this "figure" has frozen and carries with it a moral judgment about the other person. Any other data about or experience of the other is lost and seemingly unable to be accessed in the "ground."

Human beings are social beings and they respond to the context, structure and signals they are receiving. Given these seemingly insurmountable divides in our work with elected officials and the public, NICD creates safe spaces where they meet each other as human beings first. They learn about their values and important life experiences that have shaped their views before they are identified by their political labels or ideological policy positions. Thus, their "figure" of the other is completely different. Invariably they discover that they have far more in common than they could imagine. And more often than not, they discover they actually like one another and often become friends or at a minimum respectful colleagues.

In the political context this leads to action taken mutually by members of both parties to take more time to build relationships across the aisle and then to take actions to make systemic and/or structural changes in how they are working together. One of my favorite examples occurred recently in Maine. The incoming Senate President and Speaker of the House have both experienced our workshop entitled "Building Trust through Civil Discourse" and are committed to a more civil and productive legislative session.

As one important step to achieve that goal, they decided to dramatically change the seating arrangement on the floor of both chambers. Instead of the long-standing tradition of all Republicans (Rs) sitting on one side of the aisle and all Democrats (Ds) on the other, the senators and representatives are seated alternately R, D, R, D, etc. Imagine the increase in conversation and personal connection that this single structural change will lead to. Hopefully you are also recognizing the profound link between transformative change in organizations/institutions and individuals.

When you read the cases in this book you will find many specific examples of how other fundamental principles of Gestalt and systems theory – such as, presence, use-of-self, levels of system, resistance, and pragnanz – have made a profound difference in organizations in very different cultures around the world. And also, how the integration of Gestalt theory and practice into organization development can increase the reach and impact of both fields.

Brenda and Mary Ann have done the field a great service in creating this book. As a reader it makes no difference if you are new to the principles and practices of Gestalt methodology or a seasoned practitioner, the cases in this book will encourage you to step out of your comfort zone and experiment with new ways to impact systems and/or to take the next step in your own journey toward wholeness.

We are living in a time of chaotic structural change and realignment in many fundamental arenas of human activity: social, political, economic, financial, and technological. The gift we can give each other in every moment is to be fully present and engage each other with wonder and curiosity, committed to recognizing our common humanity.

A Reflection of Gestalt Practice: A Short Version of My Misunderstanding of Gestalt

Peter Block

My affection for Gestalt began sixty years ago. It took me to a weekend workshop in a barn in New Hope, Pennsylvania. It took me to Esalen Institute at Big Sur, California. Of all the different therapies I explored, it was the most efficient, brutal, to the point, and absent of analyzing the world – one of my continuing resistances to living.

So it began as a long and personal journey to make sense of my life.

Then it became the foundation of my consulting work in organization development. Whenever I was lost and had no idea what was happening, I would go around the room and ask, "How do you feel? What do you want?" I did it often enough that I wrote a book on consulting that was mostly organized around these questions. I once told a friend that I felt guilty making a living off of two questions. He said, "What else is there?"

The value of the questions is their power to value experience over intellect. The argument between science and religion is incomplete. What completes the conversation is experience. The existence of God, the empiricism of science: interesting but inconclusive. What is interesting and conclusive is that if you aspire to act on what you know, this can be found in your own body. This is the ultimate challenge of any therapy, intervention, strategic planning: "Will you act on what you know?" Gestalt is unrelenting on this question.

This is the essence of freedom, of relationship, of a fully lived life. These are central to changing organizational culture. The dominant narrative of system living is that predictability, consistency and control produce high performance. A childish myth. Mostly they produce fear, isolation and compliance.

Asking how you feel, and what you want, collectively, in a context of support is the essence of transformation. We learn and shift our thinking and our relationships with others at the citadel of our own experience, put into words in the presence of others.

If you care about transformation, or learning, or creating an organization that delivers on its promise, put best practices aside. Pay no attention to learning from history. Pay no attention to learning from your elders. Or what your precious children taught you. Pay no attention to what gives you bliss, or joy, or letting the ocean remind you of what a small and lucky being you are. These are fine comforts. So are a pillow and socks that fit. This is not cynicism. It is the expression of faith. Existential faith.

Gestalt for me is an unsentimental version of a life. It demands we accept our own human landscape. That freedom occurs when you understand that no one is watching. That understanding and judgment are the booby prizes. It ends the need for violence in its more subtle forms of self-improvement, and trying hard.

Two years ago, at the end of a workshop that I ran which went well, I declared to a participant that this experience was so different, more powerful than other groups I had led in the company. I said I wondered why? He said, "Peter, can't you just enjoy this experience, and stop trying to analyze everything?"

Evidently not.

Introduction

Mary Ann Rainey and Brenda B. Jones, Editors

Origin of this Book

It was at a conference in 2009 sponsored by NTL Institute that we began talking about a book on Gestalt. The focus of the conference was the state of the field of Organization Development (OD) and exploration of the emergence of a "new OD" paradigm (since labelled "Dialogic OD"). The conference was useful because it represented a concerted effort by OD scholars, practitioners and some of their clients to reflect on where OD has been, where it is, and increasing its future relevancy.

What stood out to us and other Gestalt practitioners at the conference was that many of the perspectives and frames of reference presented felt similar to Gestalt – developing use-of-self and presence; convening the whole system; thinking systemically, embracing diversity, inclusion and social justice; using dialogue to build collaborative and connected communities; optimism; attending to boundaries; embracing polarities and multiple realities; and re-framing the role of leadership. Of course, we were thrilled that many of the Gestalt principles we use routinely were considered important to contemporary OD practice; yet, Gestalt was never mentioned. We were not presuming that everything comes from Gestalt because we know Gestalt is a composite of many disciplines. But again, a pattern was emerging where despite the existence of a comprehensive and longstanding body of knowledge that is Gestalt, it is often not known, not recognized or not credited.

We left the conference inspired to shift this phenomenon and committed to publishing a book on Gestalt.

At its core, Gestalt is a stance – a way of being, seeing, thinking and behaving in the world. Its applicability is both timeless and boundless. The global community of Gestalt devotees see this stance as a refreshing and intriguing alternative to traditional ways of working with individuals, groups, organizations and larger systems. It serves as a useful lens through which they can view both their work life and personal life. For them, Gestalt is the embodiment of a "holistic daily operating system."

It must be acknowledged that Gestalt has challenges, some of its own making: e.g., a long history dating back to the turn of the 20st century with a protracted period with no new research and theory; association with Gestalt therapy that is sometimes misunderstood and perceived as controversial; the separation of foundational Gestalt research and theory of Kurt Lewin from the primary principles of Gestalt practice shaped by Fritz Perls; and the need of organizations and the field of organizational behavior to quickly embrace all that is shiny and new. It is often the case that the incorporation and absorption of strong, foundational ideas over time leads to a loss of distinct and unique identity. This has been the fate of Gestalt.

Still, in the face of such headwinds, Gestalt stands. In many ways, Gestalt is experiencing a 21st century resurgence. Education and training programs are growing worldwide and the number of publications is increasing. We hope this project contributes to the positive trajectory.

Objective of this Book

The overall objective of this book is two-fold: (1) to provide a practical resource for leaders, managers, administrators, consultants and other professionals on the Gestalt approach to organizational, large complex system, and leadership effectiveness and (2) encourage interest among today's organizational scholars and practitioners in expanding the body of research, theory, and practice of Gestalt.

Organization of this Book

The breadth and depth of Gestalt is represented here. The articles cover a broad spectrum of topics: philosophy, theory, concepts, and principles; spirituality, energy and behavior; working with individuals, groups, organizations and large complex systems; neuroscience; technology; coaching, leadership and change; models, tools, and strategies of application; and, use-of-self and presence. Each chapter showcases how seamlessly Gestalt principles can align with and complement current professional practice and personal life strategies.

The authors represent seven countries and confirm the global reach of Gestalt. Many have a long professional history in Gestalt. Others are early in their Gestalt journey. The combination creates innovative and provocative ideas.

The chapters are organized under four main sections:
I. Roots of Gestalt Practice
II. The Gestalt Practioner
III. Gestalt Practice at Multiple Levels of System
IV. Gestalt Approach to Change

Section One: Roots of Gestalt Practice

The introductory section, "Roots of Gestalt," establishes the foundation upon which the other three sections are built. It provides context and insight into the mindset of early Gestalt pioneers and influencers. It begins with an in-depth interview with the late Edwin C. Nevis, co-founder of the Cleveland approach to Gestalt practice in organizations and author of the classic 1987 text, *Organizational Consulting: A Gestalt Approach*. Nevis taught and mentored both of us and many of the other authors in this book.

In the next chapter, "The Relevance of Gestalt Principles and Theory," renowned scholar, author and professor W. Warner Burke addresses the significance of Gestalt therapy to OD practice.

We conclude the first section with author and Gestalt practitioner Paul Barber's "Gestalt as a Living Spiritual Practice?" where he explores Gestalt as a post-modern spiritual discipline.

Section Two: The Gestalt Practitioner

The second section focuses on the Gestalt practitioner. In her chapter entitled, "A Short Note on Use of Self and Gestalt," author and global OD trailblazer Mee-Yan Cheung-Judge traces the roots of this unique and powerful Gestalt concept and the environment from which it emerged.

In "Four Roles of the Gestalt Intervener: Holistic Presence Using Experiential Learning Theory," co-editor and behavioral scientist Mary Ann Rainey provides pragmatic intervention strategies by integrating classic Gestalt principles and contemporary research on experiential learning.

Section Three: Gestalt Practice at Multiple Levels of System

The first chapter in section three, "Navigating the Inner Emotional Landscape in a Globalized World," is contributed by international Gestalt practitioner Eva Röettgers who brings neuroscience to the discussion. The author uses Gestalt principles to understand and map the human capacity to digest the increasing complexity of our internal and external environments.

In "Preventing the Tragedy of Commons: A Call to Gestalt OD Practitioners to Pursue Holism for the Renewal of Our Global Systems," author and international OD consultant Kate Cowie explores the phenomenon of "collective renewal," drawing on the Gestalt principles of holism, general systems theory and paradoxical theory of change.

Our next chapter, "Gestalt Coaching for Awareness Management: The Elements of Mastery," offers Gestalt tools that enable coaches to heighten client awareness. Author and Gestalt therapist and consultant Dorothy E. Siminovitch believes awareness management is at the heart of Gestalt coaching and provides insights for personal and professional mastery.

Author and Gestalt practitioner Ollie Malone, Jr states that a call to adventure requires great leaders. In his chapter, "The Executive's Gestalt," Malone takes a close look at the role of leadership – what it is and how executives can improve their performance through the application of Gestalt principles.

Energy and Movement take center stage in "I'm Better When I Move: Facilitating Movement and Energy in Groups from a Gestalt Perspective" by seasoned Gestalt practitioner and group facilitator Walt Hopkins. In distinct narrative style, Hopkins takes the reader on a journey in storytelling that describes his Gestalt-based approach to energy and movement work.

Awareness also plays a central role in "The Cape Cod Model in Organizational Settings." Author and Gestalt therapist and consultant Joseph Melnick outlines a contemporary Gestalt intervention process based on positive psychology and optimism.

In the next chapter, "Gestalt Practice in Large Complex Social Systems: Communities, Clans, Tribes and Other Collective Cultural Configurations," South African coach and organizational practitioner Chantelle Wyley, explores the cultural impact of Gestalt. She helps readers see the tension Gestalt practice encounters in eliciting an "I want" in predominately "We need" cultures.

In the concluding chapter of section three, we find international Gestalt practitioner Eugenio Moliní's "Case Study: A Holistic Strategy with

Gestalt." Molini presents solutions for practitioners using a client case that reveals how Gestalt principles guided a team's process and progress after detecting counterproductive patterns and tensions.

Section Four: Gestalt Approach to Change

In opening section four, Gudrun Frank takes Gestalt into the digital world in "A Gestalt Approach to Optimizing Competence in Digital Transformation." Frank, a mechanical engineer, occupational scientist and Gestalt practitioner developed the "5 C-Model," a basic tool for optimizing competence in technology professions.

The focus shifts to the Gestalt approach to change with international organizational consultant and executive coach Jonno Hanafin's chapter, "Leading Change." His chapter presents Gestalt perspectives and models that provide powerful and practical tools for leaders who are launching, managing, and closing change initiatives.

Co-editor, author and international OD practitioner Brenda B. Jones follows with "Transformational Change Using Six C's" where she examines the process of change from both Gestalt and system perspectives. They also are foundational to the "3 C's plus 3 C's" construct she designed for transformations.

Extensive training programs have led to a steady growth of Gestalt OD practitioners in West Africa, the locus of our concluding chapter, "Cultural Underpinnings of Resistances in Organizational Change," by pastors, teachers and OD practitioners John Nkum and Dan Inkoom. Their chapter includes anecdotal evidence of the influence of Gestalt on leadership behavior and mindset from their many years of consulting practice in Ghana, Nigeria, Liberia, Sierra Leone and southern Africa.

The contributions in this book were informed by our true purpose at its beginning: to provide a useful resource on the holistic Gestalt approach and to motivate leaders, scholars and practitioners toward continuing research, theories, and practice of Gestalt. We hope you experience the book in this way.

We remain grateful for our lifelong learning and development, guided and enriched by the practice of Gestalt.

The Editors

I. ROOTS OF GESTALT PRACTICE

Chapter 1: Edwin C. Nevis Interview – The Cycle of Experience

Interview with Edwin C. Nevis, co-founder of the Gestalt-oriented management and consulting approach. Originally published in Bermann, G. & Meurer, G. (Eds.). (2000). Best Patterns – Erfolgsmuster fur Zukunftsfahiges Management, (pp. 27-31). Hemnn Luchterhand Verlag, GmbH. Neuwied und Kriftel.*

Additional information:

Ed Nevis is one of the founders of the Gestalt-oriented organizational consulting and Gestalt management approach. Gestalt therapy was developed by Laura and Fritz Perls, two German Jews, in the 1920s. They had to emigrate and, like many scientists and artists in the USA, found a new home. Ed Nevis picked up these ideas and developed them into a coherent concept.

One of the essential tools is the so-called Cycle of Experience, which is a universal process design and forms the basis of this book in the form of the learning and solution cycle. Some other methods such as figuring, working with resistance, the Unit of Work and the Levels of Systems form a holistic management and consulting concept. The contributions of Mary Ann Rainey / Claire Stratford, Paul Pape Senner, Eva and Jürgen Ferchland, as well as Lone Daalsgard / Jan Bendix are in the same tradition.

In addition to basic theoretical research, Edwin Nevis taught and researched for many years at MIT and holds a PhD in Organizational Psychology. Ed Nevis has extensive 40 years of experience advising countless well-known companies. He has also initiated and shaped a

---

* The interview was conducted on the sidelines of one of the International OSD workshops. Ed Nevis launched these programs several years ago. At this workshop, which took us to Italy, the Netherlands, Israel, Sweden and Ireland, 45 people (consultants, theorists, managers) from 20 different countries (including South Africa, Argentina, Singapore, Hungary) participated. This conversation started in Ireland and was completed "virtually". The questions were asked by Gustav Bergmann.

large international network of experts. He is co-founder of the Gestalt Institute of Cleveland and editor of the Gestalt Review. Today he is particularly involved in transcultural education and training. Personally, I have received tremendous impulses from him and have been able to experience illuminating workshops in the international field with him.

G.B.: *Gestalt Theory and Gestalt Therapy are well known concepts. Could you tell us something about the development and the "specialties" of the Gestalt OSD approach, its background and theoretical basis?*

E.N.: The application of Gestalt Therapy concepts and methods to Organization and System Development Consulting stems to a large extent from the coincidental fact that two of the early students of Fritz and Laura Perls, Isadore From, and Paul Goodman – Richard W. Wallen and I – were trained in organizational psychology, social psychology, and psychotherapy before we became involved with Gestalt Therapy in 1954. Wallen and I, working at the Gestalt Institute of Cleveland, recognized that several cornerstones of the Gestalt approach were highly applicable to organizational interventions:

The organism/environment relationship in which human processes were involved in finding out what one needed from his environment and how he went about getting it. We realized that Perls' model was a variation of system input-transformation-output models, with the individual considered to be a system made up of many parts. By simply viewing organizations as organisms, it was possible to apply Gestalt thinking at a more complex level of system with its subparts being made up of more than one individual.

- The meaning of resistance, and a way of working with it: Gestalt Therapy views resistance as a healthy phenomenon and a label placed on someone by someone on those who do not want to be influenced, and stresses the importance of working with clients' objections to a certain until these are fully understood and owned. There is a direct and immediate application of this theory to the organizational setting: when faced with resistance the strategy of those trying to implement a change is to become interested and engaged in it as a manifestation of energy directed away from that of the change agent. Wallen and I introduced this notion into management development and sensitivity training interventions and began to teach them to managers.
- Use of self as an active participant in interventions: Prior to this time management consultants were generally trained to be

more aloof and detached in dealing with their clients. Gestalt Therapy and its early proponents and teachers produced highly energized reactions in sharing their own thoughts, feelings, and observations in gnarl with their clients.
- The approach was enlarged and enhanced in the mid-1960s when a group of graduate students in the Organization Behavior Department of Case Western Reserve University came to study at the Cleveland Institute. This younger group, together with me and a psychotherapist, formed an intensive OSD Program in the mid-1970s.

G.B.: How would you explain or define leadership and management from a Gestalt Perspective?

E.N.: From a Gestalt Perspective, leadership is best seen as the use of oneself as an instrument of influence. Presence – what one has internalized and can articulate without thinking about it – is one of the most powerful ways of motivating and inspiring others. This way of thinking is consistent with theories of modeling, and with the notion of "transformational leadership" as developed by James McGregor Burns and extended by Bernard Bass. An important part of this is for the leader to be available to the followers and to work from a high-contact, rather than a detached perspective.

G.B.: What are the particular influences of Systems Theory and other approaches on Gestalt OSD and vice versa?

E.N.: Though different in some aspects, Systems Theory and the Gestalt approach are compatible. Both focus on "wholes" and "patterns and relationships" in complex settings; both are information-processing models, and both stress that actions at any system level in an organization have an impact on other parts.

A major difference is that Systems Theory focuses more on cause-effect relationships among structures and parts, and Gestalt Theory assumes a more existential position. The former frequently follows a historical analysis while the later focuses more on "here-and-now" phenomena. Another major difference is that Systems Theory tends to emphasize negative feedback – the way organisms adapt to their environment and achieve steady states – and Gestalt Theory is a growth model emphasizing positive feedback – a process of change that expands possibilities. Of course, new thinking about chaos theory and self-organizing systems is moving Systems Theory and Gestalt Theory closer together.

G.B.: The Gestalt Cycle of Experience is a fundamental tool and it helps us to create useful process designs. How do you use it in your work? Please explain how it leads to contact.

E.N.: The Cycle of Experience is a way of conceptualizing the fundamental human process of finding out what you need (awareness), mobilizing for action to obtain it (making contact), and learning from the experience (making meaning out of it). It is useful in several ways. First, it provides a useful guideline in assessing where the client is at any moment and to determine whether to support more data-gathering (awareness) or to encourage movement into action. Frequently, it tells the intervener that a group is moving too quickly into action and acting on limited data in its zeal to get something accomplished. By using this lens, the intervener can direct his or her efforts more precisely. A second use is for interveners to apply to themselves. Are they grounding themselves by getting enough data before they move ahead? This use is similar to performing organizational assessments or doing survey interventions. These allow interveners to position themselves to do their work.

G.B.: Sometimes it is hard to balance the need of content and the necessity of managing the process. How could the Gestalt approach help to balance content and process?

E.N.: The Gestalt model is a process model. It provides a way for practitioners to work well with almost any content. Information technologists, architects, environmental consultants, and others can use the concepts and methods to enhance their work in influencing the client to respond more fully to their technical services. For example, I have applied the Gestalt approach in such areas as changing a poorly functioning incentive compensation. In this instance I initiated a look at this system, and together with a compensation specialist, designed and influenced acceptance of a new system. I used my process skills, but combined these with content inputs concerning motivational theory and performance management systems.

G.B.: In the New Economy more and more people feel lost in "cyber space". The companies lose corporate identity and cohesion. How can we reestablish contact, connection, and understanding in a virtual and digital economy? What are the common rules, issues, shared visions to which we can refer to in a social system?

E.N.: I believe that much can be accomplished in "cyber space" if it involves communication among people who know each other and who can meet face-to-face from time to time. Personally, I am very suspicious of "instant connections" via the Internet. We have too many examples of people manipulating others or of "instant relationships" that have gone wrong because insufficient common groundwork did not allow for true contact. A psychiatrist has written about this, making a strong case for what he called "human moments". Even teleconferencing – that at least lets people see each other – does not provide for a full taking in of the other person.

However, if I know someone through face-to-face experiences, I can use mental pictures of that person while we are communicating electronically.

Secondly, I believe that corporate identity and confusion may occur due to over-communication as well as under-communication. If I receive a constant stream of messages nothing will stand out and I will pay less attention to the messages. As in many things, "less is more" in cyberspace.

G.B.: Many years ago you founded the international OSD workshop. As a member of the fourth program I had the opportunity to experience the fundamental differences of culture. How would you explain the concept of multiple realities and the importance of cultural differences in a global economy?

E.N.: The concept of alternate or varying realities stems from several phenomenological theories. Basically, it says that people occupying the same space and witnessing a presumably common event will have different experiences. An accountant will think of salespersons' expenses as costs to be controlled; the salesperson will see it as an investment in obtaining future business. Kurt Lewin said that "every child is born into a different family", implying that siblings make meaning out of their family experience in different ways. Some years ago, in order to find a way of eliminating the word "resistance" – which has very negative connotations and is a label that one puts on another who does not want to go where he is driving – I proposed that we think of this as a matter of "multiple realities", and that we accept both of these as valid perceptions. This enables the agent of change to become interested in both his and the other's sides, rather than to dismiss the other. One of the reasons why this Gestalt concept has proven very powerful in multicultural work is that it assumes that all cultures have valid and useful premises and assumptions. Each represents another reality and to be successful in cross-cultural work requires tolerance and understanding of one's own and the other's culture. The underlying assumption is that of tolerance of differences, as opposed to being righteous in favor of one's own. Absorbing this stance has made it possible for me to work successfully in all corners of the world, and this is what I try to inculcate in my students. As someone who studied with me, you can comment on this better than I can.

G.B.: Where do you see the future trends of Gestalt OSD?

E.N.: I believe that the next application of the Gestalt approach will be at the community level, as opposed to the organizational level. This has already been started, and we will see more of it. By community I mean a broader association of people with a common interest, such as a group of firms in an alliance; a housing community, a group of the various stakeholders in a given local who are concerned with and or deliver health services, the members of a given profession, etc. This level is more responsive to the actuality of the current world; the boundaries among entities are more fluid than ever before in history. If I were younger, I would attempt to move my practice to this level. While there are many practical issues, such as how to determine what a given community is, how to get the various parts to meet, and who would pay for my services, this is the direction of the future.

G.B.: Around the Gestalt Institute of Cleveland you have initiated and organized a network and community. Please tell us something about your plans and activities.

E.N.: I have a natural inclination to create networks and communities. I am now working on putting together two networks, one for Gestalt-oriented teaching and publishing ventures, and one for self-organized, peer-group continuous learning by faculty and graduates of major training institutes. Both of these networks will be truly international in character, with coordinating offices in the US, Europe, and Israel. And they will bring clinically- and organizationally-oriented practitioners under one umbrella. The networks will be supported by the Gestalt International Study Center, a kind of R&D organization that I created in 1979.

G.B.: Gestalt Therapy was founded by two German Jews, Laura and Fritz Perls, who had to emigrate in the 1930s. During our international program we met each other in Jerusalem. For me as a German it was a healing process to work in Israel with Jewish people in a multicultural context. I felt accepted and respected. And I think it has a lot to do with your approach and facilitation. it was a journey from feeling guilt towards responsibility. Could you please tell us how we can reduce all kinds of racism and discrimination in our daily work as consultants. Is there something like a Gestalt ethic or imperative?

E.N.: I think I addressed this above. I do not know whether there is a Gestalt ethic or imperative, but I do know that you cannot teach or influence others until you are willing to deal with your own racism or sexism. This works in all directions. As a Jew, I had very negative stereotypes about Germans and an understandable aversion to working with Germans or going to Germany. I was finally persuaded in 1988 by some Jewish colleagues who had worked in Germany that a German post-WWII generation was quite different from my images of the holocaust would lead me to believe.

Only by working with individual Germans and seeing their humanity and the price they paid as children of Nazi-era parents could I begin to come close to any kind of forgiveness, or at least to see my German students as individuals. From my experience in trying to deal with my feelings, I developed a sense of how to facilitate relationships between Germans and Jews. As you know, I put groups together in which there are many different cultures, but always some Germans and Israelis, and I have taken these groups both to Germany and to Israel. I think that I was aided in doing this by 40 years of experience in working cross-culturally.

G.B.: Thank you Edwin.

References

Nevis, E. (1988) Organizational Consulting. Cambridge, MA: Gestalt Institute of Cleveland Press.

Nevis, E., DiBella, A. J. (1998) *How Organizations Learn*. San Francisco: Jossey Bass.

Nevis, E., Lancourt, J., Vasallo, H. (1996) *Intentional Revolutions*. San Francisco: Jossey Bass.

Chapter 2: The Relevance of Gestalt Therapy Principles and Theory to Organization Development Consultation

W. Warner Burke

The purpose of this chapter is to show the relevance of Gestalt therapy to organization development (OD) practice. A number of Gestalt principles are covered with case examples to provide applicability to OD consultative practice. We begin with an OD case that was a failure followed by "correctives" that build on "better OD" but also the relevance and applicability of Gestalt principles. The paper consists of two parts – the failure case with correctives and a second part that emphasizes human energy from a Gestalt perspective.

The Case
It is possible to fail in many ways....
While to succeed is possible only in one way
(for which reason also one is easy and the other difficult
– to miss the mark easy, to hit it difficult).

Aristotle
384-322 B.C.

Occasionally an external consultant will be asked by the client to join their organization on a fulltime basis. Such was the case circa 1972 with Stephen Fuller who was a Harvard Business School professor and had been consulting with General Motors for a number of years. GM wanted him to join their executive ranks and serve as head of the human resource function, what today we would call the Chief Human Resource Officer and a member of the C-suite. Although Fuller's background was in organizational behavior and employee relations, relevant to HR, he had not been a corporate executive before. By 1974 Fuller decided that he could use some help from someone like his former self – an external consultant. I was contacted by his office to see if I would be interested in serving in such a role. After all, they said, Chris Argyris had recommended me. I was thrilled and immediately said "yes, I will be happy to serve." General Motors was #1 on the Fortune 500 list at the time. This was "heady stuff." After our initial meeting and reaching some agreement about how we would work together, it was clear to me that I liked Steve and wanted him to succeed. But succeed at what? It ever so gradually became obvious to me that he and I were not on the same page about what success looked like. For me success was running a high-performance HR function, that is, to lead and manage his people in an empowering manner and applying the latest evidence for what effective HR operations should be. Also I wanted to help him develop his management group into a high performing team. Steve had other things in mind. To my surprise he was very much a political animal managing across and upward. For example, when we had lunch together in the executive dining room (yes, there were private dining rooms for top executives in those days.), Steve would rarely look at me sitting across the table from him; rather, he would be scanning the room to see who was dining with whom and wondering what they might be talking about. Try as I might I could not get him to lead the HR function nor to spend any significant time building his team. Steve spent his time relating with his fellow executives and the CEO. How he spent his time and energy had some degree of payoff. He was at GM in that capacity for about 11 years. I do not remember exactly but my time there was not much more than 11 months. I simply had no influence on him.

I am usually hard on myself regarding my work and this time I felt that I had failed. To simplify, overly so I suspect, I knew that I could facilitate team building in my sleep. I grew up on group dynamics – the T Group and process consultation. I was educated as a social psychologist meaning interpersonal and group relations. But when it came to one-on-one consulting, what today we call executive coaching, I considered myself to be inadequate. I decided then and there that I must do something about my inadequacy. I had heard about the Gestalt therapy training program at the Cleveland Institute. Two of my friends who knew me well had attended the eight-week program held annually for 13 months. I asked each one independently whether he thought the program would be a good fit for me. Both said absolutely, because there was a total system approach which fit my taste perfectly and the staff were outstanding. I signed up. My intent was not to conduct therapy, rather to become more effective as a consultant in a one-on-one setting, that is, executive coaching. My job was to apply the therapeutic learning to a consulting situation. Ever since, the mid 70s, I have been grateful for what I learned and subsequently have applied.

Armed with Gestalt therapy subsequent to the GM venture what might I have done differently in my work with Steve Fuller? At least seven "corrections" come to mind some directly from my Gestalt experience and some from better OD in general. The Gestalt points to be made, and noted as we proceed, come from my memory and what I believe I have learned. In other words, I deliberately did *not* go to my notes, articles, and books from the training I received. I wanted to see what has stuck with me, has become second nature to my consulting work. These points are noted in italics. But the first of my seven corrections is from OD in general not from Gestalt therapy as such yet there is relevance to Gestalt therapy.

1. **Contracting**: Clearly I was not sufficiently clear about an agreement with Fuller in terms of how we would work together. Weisbord's (1973) wonderful article had just been published in the *OD Practitioner* and provided the necessary and important ingredients of OD contracting. I don't remember but apparently I took Weisbord's advice for granted and didn't pay adequate attention to goals, Fuller's role compared with mine, timelines, mutual expectations, and related matters. What I know now with a great deal of certainty regarding OD contracting are (a) when things go wrong in the consultant-client relationship it means that our original contracting was faulty or changed due to circumstances beyond our control and must be corrected, and (b) that contracting is practically a constant process. Each meeting with the client should begin with at least a quick review of "where we are" in our working relationship compared with what we have agreed to in the past, even if the past is only last week. Unplanned change occurs so rapidly these days we can easily miss important consequences to our original agreement that make a difference and therefore at least a "tweaking" to our contract is necessary to ensure effective work together.

2. **The Larger System-Context**: Gestalt thinking is all about the total system. A goal of therapy is to integrate more effectively disparate parts of the total person, e.g., unresolved issues in one's life. My client, Fuller, was part of a larger system. My job was to gain information about his larger system, and while I interviewed his subordinates I did not speak with his peers nor his boss, the CEO. These were the people he was paying most attention to not his direct reports. I tried to obtain significant information about how Fuller was perceived by these others and what pressures he may have been experiencing from them. I was trying to work on his team rather than the team where he

was a member not the boss. To state the obvious, I missed understanding critical information about the larger system and where Fuller was organizationally and politically in that broader context. It may have been, for example, that the CEO wanted more from Fuller as an advisor to him than for him to spend a lot of time on running the HR function. I had an inappropriate perspective due to my not learning about the larger system and Fuller's role and function within it.

3. **Fields of Forces**: As we know Kurt Lewin was originally trained in Gestalt psychology. (Gestalt is a German word for which there is no direct translation in English. We assume "pattern" or "whole" may be the closest meaning.) Lewin's theory was primarily based on physics, however. Thus, he viewed a given human situation as one influenced by "fields of forces". These forces differed with respect to intensity and therefore have different affects on the human being, some pushing a person in one direction and some restraining the person from acting. It is likely in addition to the influence of physics Lewin viewed a situation in its totality, that is, from a Gestalt perspective. In any case, two points are highly relevant for OD consultation. First, one of our most powerful tools is the force field analysis and with respect to change is always relevant, i.e., what forces are driving change yet at the same time what other forces are restraining, creating barriers for change. For the classic example of this point see the Coch and French study (1948) which shows how driving and restraining forces affect productivity in a manufacturing plant. Second, and overlapping with the first point, as consultants we want to know what pressures at work the client is experiencing. A central concept in Gestalt therapy is *energy* the theme of the second part of this paper. How does the client spend his or her energy at work? Responding to pressures requires energy. Knowing how organizational members spend their time, and what pressures they experience is diagnostically very important. I don't recall ever asking Fuller what pressures he felt. Showing a bit of empathy on my part might have helped. Knowing more about the forces impinging on him every day and the overall pressures of the business in the automotive marketplace at the time would no doubt have helped me to be more relevant rather than puzzled about why I was having no influence on Fuller. These two points recognize the importance in OD consultation of combining field theory and the Gestalt principle of how energy is spent.

4. **Resistance**: Inherent within the concept of *resistance* is energy – a clenched fist, a tight jaw, and/or a stubborn point of view that is difficult if not impossible to forego. Why, then, a separate section on resistance? First, most people believe that when it comes to change, resistance is inevitable and therefore must be confronted and dissipated. In other words, resistance is intrinsic to change. Second, resistance is not as simple as the first reason implies. Resistance is not always the response to change and what appears to be resistance may be something else. Almost two decades ago, Piderit (2000) argued persuasively that what may be perceived as resistance could actually be nothing more than ambivalence. The proposed change might be perceived as the right thing to do but one is simply not sure. Such questioning can be seen as resistance but for the change consultant a more persuasive argument is required not one form of resistance facing another. Moreover, when resistance is for real it is rarely the change itself that is the culprit, but rather it is the imposition of change that is resisted. In Gestalt therapy the therapist sees resistance to change by the patient as a significant diagnostic. It often concerns something that the patient is holding on to, not willing to let go – a failed marriage, loss of a job, some habitual process that seems to hurt rather than help the patient, etc. Thus, resistance can be a refusal to let go of the past. The work of William Bridges (1980) can be quite useful under these circumstances. His simple yet eloquent three-phase model regarding change can be helpful – letting go –transitioning – new beginnings. One cannot transition to a changed condition unless the individual lets go of the past. The model is also appropriate at the group and organizational levels. Resistance therefore is a particular form of how *energy* is used. Discovering that use, for example, how my client, Fuller, spent his time, is critical to bringing about change. Holding on to the past – a particular belief, a way of doing things – requires energy. Releasing that energy in new directions is a form of change.

5. **Wants**: A, perhaps the, fundamental question a Gestalt therapist asks the patient and continues to ask over many sessions is "What do you *want*?" What do you want to happen regarding the issue being confronted and discussed? What do you want us to address, to dig into over the next hour? These *want* questions are relevant for a group and at the organizational level, and may sound obvious. Isn't it about a

goal or objective? Yes, but the change consultant with the question must reach the emotional level. The question concerns motivation, desire, being realistic and perhaps helping to understand why the person, the group, is stuck seemingly unable to address new issues and possibilities. If memory serves, my client, Fuller, avoided any discussion of feelings like the plague, and I did not confront that avoidance to the degree that I should have.

6. **Managing Time**: In organization change work as in Gestalt therapy *time* is a precious commodity. There never seems to be enough time to do what needs to be done. In Gestalt therapy the present is the primary focus, the here and now, not the past, and if we manage the present well, the future will more or less take care of itself. Not that the past is ignored; its relevance concerns how the past affects the issue at hand. The past cannot be managed; the present can. This point relates to the previous notion of "letting go." In addition to a focus on the present, a principle of Gestalt therapy is recognition of the passage of time between sessions with the therapist and the patient (client). The beginning of session two (or three or twelve) is never something like, "Now let's see, where did we leave off from our last session?" Nor, "What do we need to continue from our last meeting?" Events happen in between sessions. The start of each session therefore begins with the present not last week or last month. The question is something like "How are you feeling now? What's on your mind? What are you feeling good about at the moment? What are you not feeling so good about?" In other words, each session is a present analysis that deals with the patient's current concerns. In most respects these Gestalt therapy principles apply to organization change consulting. The client is never where he or she was when we last worked together. The passage of time these days is often referred to as "warp speed."
I would like to think that I conformed to these principles when working with my client at GM. I honestly cannot remember. It was a long time ago and much has happened regarding my development since 1974. But that time with Fuller was before my training in Gestalt therapy so the odds are that I did not pay adequate attention to the passage of time and what was happening within those passages.

7. **Covert Processes**: When working with patients and clients, of utmost importance in both Gestalt therapy and organization

change consultation is not just what the patient or client says but what is not said. This final "corrective" point is more applicable to groups than individuals yet in a one-on-one context collusion can occur where there is some implicit agreement about what is "on the table" and what is not. To some extent there was collusion between Fuller and myself in that what was never overtly addressed was that we had separate agendas. My agenda concerned his leadership of the HR function, and his agenda was about his influence laterally and upward within the C suite. Fuller, of course, could have been more explicit about what he wanted from me, but to my knowledge he had never been a client before and he may have assumed that it was my responsibility as the consultant to discern what was needed. And I could have worked much more with him about his agenda in terms of interviewing his peers and boss and explaining what I saw as the group dynamics, overt and covert, of the C-suite members, i.e., what were their collusions and how he might influence them. Had I been more astute at the time, I could have used psychodynamic theory, group-as-a-whole level analysis, and social structure concepts (Noumair, 2013) to help Fuller understand his role and his own susceptibility to collusion.

With this final "corrective" I have begun to move beyond Gestalt therapy theory and dabble in the psychodynamic arena with Freud vs. Fritz Perls all over again. But the point is we need both to understand more fully the complex aspects of human behavior. Allow me to stop here and not fuel the differences between Gestalt psychology and psychodynamic theory. Besides I have found both to be valuable and helpful in identifying a more complete whole, or a Gestalt if you will, of human nature.

Human Energy
Energy in the Executive is a leading character in the definition of good government.

Alexander Hamilton, The New York Packet, Tuesday, March 18, 1788.

One of my primary mentors for OD, as is no doubt true for many of us, was Richard Beckhard particularly in the late 1960s when I was on a steep learning curve. He had a "nose" for power in organizations, who had power, how it was deployed, and whether corrupted or close to its corruption. Dick seemed to know the answers to these questions in a matter of an hour or so with the client. I never ceased to be impressed. Power was therefore his number one diagnostic. I learned a lot about power from him and rely on what he taught me to this day. But power is more like my number 2 diagnostic. Paying attention to how *human energy* is used in the workplace is number 1 for me. I consider time to be our most precious commodity. Thus, how do organizational members use their time on the job? Do people waste time?

In the early days of Jack Welch's tenure as CEO of General Electric he launched a corporate-wide change initiative that was labeled "Work Out". He authorized local managers periodically to meet with their people in small groups, with facilitators, to discuss openly and honestly what they were doing on a daily basis that they considered unnecessary, a bureaucratic process that prevented efficiency, and in general, a waste of time. Welch admonished them to "toss them out". Over time it seemed clear that "work out" led to improved productivity. My kind of classic OD intervention!

My penchant, my Beckhard nose, for how human energy is used in organizations without doubt came from my Gestalt therapy training. Gestalt therapists pay considerable attention to how patients use their energy. I have chosen three Gestalt therapy ideas, concepts, or principles to illustrate how human energy is considered and used to pursue holism. These human energy principles with case examples are:
- experimentation – the act of releasing new energy
- unfinished business – where we spend undue energy on attempting to reach closure even though this objective consistently eludes us
- integration – where disparate parts drain energy from the whole

Experimentation

At one of the evening sessions during my training at the Gestalt Institute, I was confronted by the group therapist. She thought that I had been "hanging back" in previous sessions and now it was my turn. I accepted the challenge and decided to work on a certain aspect of myself that had both been of benefit and at times a problem – my "counter dependency". I was raised in the Deep South by a religious family with clear rules of conduct. Moreover, my dad drilled into me the importance of being independent, to "stand on my own two feet", to make it on my own, never accept a handout, and never assume that someone else will take care of me. I was the first of three children in the family and my dad wanted me to be an example, role model, for my younger brother and sister. As soon as I was old enough to have a social security card and number, at the age of 14, I needed to have a job, at least a part-time one. My dad helped me to get my first job (after that, of course, I was on my own) at Piggly Wiggly sacking groceries for customers. My first paycheck was not a check; it was cash in a brown envelope amounting to 20 or so dollars. I have received a paycheck of one form or the other for the rest of my life, i.e., standing on my own two feet. Being dependent on anyone else has been antithetical to my existence; the thought of dependency is a scary one. My fierce independence and at times counter dependency has not always been a good thing. It has on occasion led me to be obstinate, antiauthoritarian, and although rare, even rebellious. Ever so gradually I began to think that being counter dependent was not always the best route for my behavior, beliefs, and values to take. I therefore came to the conclusion that the Gestalt Institute was a safe place for me to experiment with my deepest feelings, in this case the forbidden feeling of dependency.

In my therapy group I had established a rewarding relationship with one of the men, a chaplain at a prominent university. He was a big, burly type with a teddy-bear quality. I asked him if I could curl up in his lap and otherwise he simply hold me; nothing else was required. He smiled, readily agreed, and held me for about 20 or so minutes. The therapist in the meantime worked with others in the group. When I returned to my place in the group I felt warm all over even to the point of seeming to have a fever. I could not articulate much of anything and the therapist did not push me to do so. It was all about feeling not cognition. I went to bed that night, continuing to feel feverish, and tossed and turned. The next morning I was in a group with Elaine Kepner serving as our therapist. (God bless her memory!) I asked her to help me understand what had happened, a further dependency plea as it were. Elaine explained that what I had done was to unleash a torrent of new energy in my body causing a temporary fever. And with the passing of time and reflection, I became clearer about what it all meant. Elaine was right. I have gained a deeper understanding of this kind of need. I can be dependent on others even though at times it still feels disconcerting and unsettling. And my counter dependency has largely been put to rest.

How does this personal change now affect my work as a consultant and executive coach? First, I am in a better position to coach counter-dependent executives, to help them see more clearly the consequences of unduly confronting their bosses. I can tell them my own story of having done so when I blew the whistle on my boss and was fired – see Burke (2015). Second, I can testify to the fact that experimenting on occasion can help to find new ways of operating when one feels stuck and unclear about what to do. One may not need a therapist in order to experiment, but a competent executive coach can help.

The broader point is that with change new energy in the system is released. And, finally, when OD is practiced appropriately change recipients participate in making decisions that directly affect their contributions to the change effort in particular, and their degree of engagement in general. This increase in participation typically leads to feelings of being more in control and of having more power as a part of the larger system. The astute OD practitioner will exploit in the best sense of the word, this new flush of energy to support and expedite the change effort.

Unfinished Business

Although by no means limited to Gestalt therapy the principle of unfinished business is nevertheless central to the work. Considerable time is devoted to dealing with activities and memories from the past that reside in the present, feelings that are unresolved whether we are fully conscious of them or not. These unresolved issues drain energy from us that we could otherwise use for perhaps more important purposes.

It may be that some guru in China or India centuries ago made note of the importance of unfinished business but academically we probably learned about the idea for the first time as late as the 1930s. A Russian psychologist Bluma Zeigarnik, went to Germany during that time to conduct research and study with Kurt Lewin. In a series of studies she found activities and feelings that were not completed or resolved for people were much more readily recalled than those activities that they considered completed, resolved, over and done with, as we say. This difference in recall was dubbed the "Zeigarnik effect", i.e., incomplete tasks and unresolved feelings are more easily remembered than those that were essentially completed and resolved. A few years ago I used the idea to admonish OD practitioners to tackle some unresolved issues in our field of OD (Burke, 2011). The point is that when there is unfinished business in our lives we tend to spend energy in attempts to finish what is unfinished, to achieve closure. It seems to be a basic need. Regarding highly significant events in our lives, as hard as we may try, we probably never achieve full closure. But funerals are important because they do provide an avenue for some degree of closure.

Even though it was not a funeral, I did participate in an exercise in my Gestalt therapy training that helped me considerably to achieve some degree of closure on a significant piece of unfinished business in my life at the time. A year or so prior to my training at the Institute in Cleveland and in my final year (as it turned out) as a full time professional staff member at the National Training Laboratories (NTL), I had become concerned about what I considered to be inappropriate leadership on the part of the NTL president (I was his # 2). In fact Chris Argyris an active member of the Board visited with me in private about his own concerns. The consequences of our meeting was to call an emergency Board meeting with the professional staff in attendance and for me to express my concerns, "to spill the beans," to blow the whistle, as it were. I did so and the eight-member Board was split about what to do. Two weeks later the president of NTL fired me. For two years I was on my own as an independent consultant, and at the same time, hanging on to unresolved feelings. At one of the sessions later at the Gestalt Institute, the therapist for my group was Joseph Zinker. He knew about my situation and suggested that "we work on it". Under Zinker's direction I designated roles for my fellow group participants to undertake Board members, professional staff, and of course the NTL president. Zinker then told me "to have it out with them" which I proceeded to do – yelling at them for abandoning me, telling the president he was incompetent, and accusing the Board of waffling. I vented as much rage as I could muster without physically hurting any of my fellow participants. They were terrific incidentally yelling back at me and putting me in my place. After settling down, Zinker suggested that I answer two questions: (1) What had I given to NTL over my eight-year time period as a fulltime professional staff member, and (2) what had NTL given to me? Those two questions elicited very powerful feelings including tears – feelings of gratefulness, pride, significant learning, and relief. To learn more about Zinker's work as a consummate Gestalt therapist see his book (Zinker, 1977). The activity went a long way toward my being able to let go, the importance of Phase 1 in the William Bridges (1980) model of transitions. Moreover, I gained considerable confidence in the importance of closure especially in times of change – personal and organizational. But let me quickly add that we rarely if ever achieve complete closure. The fact that I can still tell my whistle blowing story with as much detail as I have demonstrated means that my closure, while helpful, is not complete. Also the story is at the individual level. Let us now consider an example at the organizational level.

The experimental learning and increased confidence that followed from the NTL experience led me some years later to suggest a "funeral" for an expired rocket program at the Glenn Research Center of the National Aeronautics and Space Administration (NASA). The program of some 20 years had come to an end but this reality was hard to accept by the engineers and technicians involved for all of that time. But the change was "a given".

Before taking on a new program and having to acquire some new knowledge and learn new skills, senior management conducted a brief ceremony. On the front lawn in front of the administration building, a table draped in black cloth was the focal point. Underneath the cloth was a small replica of the old rocket. After the table was uncovered, certain senior managers made very brief speeches extolling the former program and the people who had contributed to it over the years. All drank a toast, and the rocket was then covered again, symbolically buried. The head of the organization then gave a short explanation of the new program (solar energy for propulsion in space) that was replacing the old. The entire event took less than 30 minutes. Accomplished with this event were two important outcomes: First, an unequivocal symbolic act demonstrated the end of the program, and second, affirmative recognition was provided for those who had been involved (Burke & Noumair, 2015; p. 193).

The head of the Center told me months later that he was convinced the burial ceremony made a difference. People had stopped asking him questions about the former rocket program of some 20 years. The ceremony helped to achieve closure on business that had not been finished.

Integration

Recall that the term Gestalt translates roughly as "whole" or "pattern". Taking a therapeutic perspective means to view the patient as a whole, the total human being. In so doing the therapist is looking for parts of the person that may be disparate, unintegrated. An obvious example might be a war veteran who has lost part of his body, say, an arm or leg. The therapeutic process is therefore focused on dealing with this reality and the acceptance of and adjustment to an artificial limb. The unintegrated part could of course be more psychological not altogether physical, for example, dealing with feedback from others that is not accepted by the patient such as being perceived as abrasive, arrogant, and intimidating. The therapist's goal may be to help the patient develop a new whole by integrating what has been a separate, unacceptable, and unintegrated part that when integrated redefines the whole; in this example, accepting the dark side of one's personality.

But let us focus more on the organizational level, a complicated process of integration for sure. A case example should help. I worked with British Airways for 5 years in the late 1980s to help with their change from a government sponsored organization to a private, stock-owned corporation. The change was sweeping, from mission and strategy, to leadership, to deeply cultural. Every level, role, and employee was directly affected – except one. Although aware of most everything that was going on, the engineering function was not touched, not directly involved in the change effort. This part of BA was primarily responsible for maintenance of the entire fleet of aircraft, a sizeable and naturally a highly important operation. Fortunately for BA this function had a stellar record of performance. BA had one of if not the best safety record in the industry. Moreover, the BA engineering function was sought after to perform on a contractual basis maintenance services for other airlines. This additional work was a significant source of income for BA. But not enough. BA was in the red financially year after year, and Margaret Thatcher, the Prime Minister, had lost all patience and declared that the airline, the "flagship" airline for the country, had to make it on their own nevertheless. The engineering function could help BA make it by operating pretty much as they had been doing for years. Their track record was for all to see. Since engineering was the bedrock of the company the change decision was to leave them alone. This decision was made ("was taken" as the British would say) for two reasons: (1) Why change this part of the BA organization if no need was seen to warrant such action? (2) An important principle of organization change is for change recipients to be clearly informed about both what will be the focus of change and what will not. In the midst of change and the consequent chaos – or "mess in the middle" – it is just as important to understand what will not change as it is important to understand what will. Change recipients need an anchor to hold on to in order to help them deal with all the machinations of any organizational change effort.

Yet the engineering function was not sufficiently integrated into the overall change process. In the spirit of integration we therefore made certain that moving forward whatever all the other changes might be, and there were many, the number one goal and central to the mission of BA was *safety*. Keeping the airplanes well-maintained was paramount.

Even though engineering was not integrated at the outset of the change effort they became a significant part of the whole with their safety responsibility. BA today remains one of the safest airlines in the world. For a more complete story of the change at BA, see Burke (2018a).

Some Final Thoughts

Organization change work is too complicated to be left to OD practitioners alone to figure it all out. Seeking a deeper understanding about change from one of our nearest neighbors, Gestalt theory and therapy, makes good sense, for example, we start from the same base – open system theory. Other examples of neighbors to learn from and expand our OD practice include social network analysis, talent management, leader development theory and research, and new forms of organizational strategy and structure such as platform organizations (think Facebook, Uber, etc.); see Burke (2018b) and Church and Burke (2017).

This journey of touching the interface of OD and Gestalt therapy has been in many respects highly personal. I didn't plan for it to be; it just seemed to happen. Which may be a commentary on how Gestalt therapy transpires – it simply emerges. I did plan to write about the GM case of failure and Stephen Fuller, however, I have written about failure before (Noumair, Winderman & Burke, 2010), although not that much. I think we should write about failure more than we do. There is much to learn. But it is embarrassing. Looking back on it, I have asked, "How could I have been so naïve, so oblivious?" Moreover, reporting on this case is an obvious example of unfinished business for me. If you, the reader, learned anything, or at least were reminded of some important issues from my failure, like the importance, of contracting, and recontracting, incorporating the larger system into the consulting process, etc., then I can live more easily with my embarrassment.

And, finally, a thought about the significance of continuous learning – regardless of age and degree of experience. When considering our professional and personal development our checklist should not be a list of skills and abilities necessarily. Rather, the focus needs to be on levels: individual, interpersonal, group, intergroup, organizational (which could be a network), and inter-organizational (think acquisition or merger). What are the requisite skill sets for each level? When first entering the field of OD, I knew some things about the individual level (training and development primarily), interpersonal, e.g., importance of delivering feedback to another person so that it can be heard, and group dynamics – norms, collusion, goals, climate, etc. Where I needed the most work was at the organizational and inter-organizational levels. And I had overlooked highly important skills at the individual level- executive coaching. Considering skill sets by level should help with organizing our thoughts and plans for where and when to focus our consulting energy and abilities.

References

Bridges, W. (1980). *Transitions*: *Making sense of life's changes*. Reading, MA: Addison-Wesley.

Burke, W.W. (2018a). *Organization change*: *Theory and practice* (5th Ed.). Thousand Oaks, CA: Sage.

Burke, W.W. (2018b). The rise and fall of organization development inventiveness. What now? *Consulting Psychology Journal*, In press.

Burke, W.W. (2015). Choice points: The making of a scholar-practitioner: In A.B. Shani & D.A. Noumair (Eds.). *Research in organizational change and development* (pp. 1-38). Bingley, U.K.: Emerald Group Publishing Ltd.

Burke, W.W. (2011). A perspective on the field of organization development and change: The Zeigarnik effect. *Journal of Applied Behavioral Science*, 47, 143–167.

Burke, W.W. & Noumair, D.A. (2015). *Organization development*: *A process of learning and changing*, 3rd Ed. Upper Saddle River, NJ: Pearson Education.

Church, A.H. & Burke, W.W. (2017). Four trends shaping the future of organizations and organization development. *OD Practitioner*, 49 (3), 14-22.

Coch, L. & French, J.R.P. (1948). Overcoming resistance to change. *Human Relations*, 1, 512-532.

Noumair, D.A. (2013). Cultural revelations: Shining a light on organizational dynamics. *International Journal of Group Psychotherapy*, 63, 153-176.

Noumair, D.A., Winderman, B.B., & Burke, W.W. (2010). Transforming the A.K. Rice Institute: From club to organization. *Journal of Applied Behavioral Science*, 46, 473-499.

Piderit, S.K. (2000). Rethinking resistance and recognizing ambivalence. A multidimensional view of attitudes toward an organizational change. *Academy of Management Review*, 25, 783-794.

Weisbord, M.R. (1973). The organization development contract. *OD Practitioner*, 5(2), 1-4.

Zinker, J. (1977). *Creative process in Gestalt therapy*. New York: Brunner/Mazel Publishers.

Chapter 3: Gestalt as a Living Spiritual Practice?

Paul Barber

Introduction

In this chapter Gestalt is suggested to be a post-modern spiritual discipline. Its illumination of the moment and robust awareness raising have much in common with other spiritual traditions. Born from out of a countercultural Humanistic womb it has sadly lost its way as a movement and become merely another psychotherapeutic method. Professionalisation is seen to have speeded this process. A reversal of this slide to conservatism and rekindling of its Humanistic origin and Zen-like spiritual nature is suggested to be necessary for its continued psychic survival. The writing style attempts to honour Gestalt, with awareness heightening questions rather than seasoned intellectual argument.

Paradoxically, its references look back to go forward!

Gestalt – Holistic Inquiry into the Essence of Being?

The transpersonal principles underpinning Gestalt have always been with us. Awareness and mindfulness beloved of Buddhism, attentiveness to bodily energy and practical experimentation cultivated by Taoism, opening to the unknown and unknowable favoured by Shamanistic traditions, exploding through the impasse of Zen – all are present. So what is different? All are woven to Humanism in service of an holistic dialogical inquiry.

If Gestalt had not been so firmly bridled to Psychotherapy it would likely have evolved into a mystical path, for it encapsulates the very essence of mindful contemplation. Indeed, its 'psychotherapeutic role' may be robbing it of its core value as a practical spiritual guide for everyday living. Fritz Perls openly acknowledged his indebtedness to Zen (Perls, 1972). Actually, Joseph Zinker observed of Gestalt's founding father:

> *"What hasn't survived about Fritz – is his presence. He was like a Zen master who taught you by... smearing himself all over you, in the most powerful way. He made you sit up"* (Zinker interviewed by Barber 2001, .p30).

Gestalt keeps us in dialogue with what is transcendent alongside what we see, feel and touch. It attends to the whole energetic field, conscious and unconscious, presence and being, past and present and imagined future. We believe that change occurs when 'what is present' is fully lived – which itself opens up another way to enlightenment (Wheway 1999, p.123). To do this we develop a thick description of our lived experiential reality until we can virtually smell and taste it. As 'all and everything' is in the field of awareness, so drawing attention to 'all and everything' is what we do. Note, those obstacles on the path to self-actualisation we highlight are the same ones that frustrate spiritual development, namely ignorance, ego, desire and attachment, hatred, anger and fear.

Some years ago I catalogued five major orientations to reality that emerged in my work with clients:

Reflecting upon Physical-Sensory Phenomenon: *[Gathering and attending to sensory information – developing sensory intelligence]* Observing and listening; attending to the environment; focusing upon what is presented; identifying physical support systems; differentiating between thoughts and feelings and observations; developing awareness and sensitivity to our physiological needs.

Reflecting upon Social-Cultural Phenomenon: *[Relating and understanding the cultural context – developing social intelligence]* Appreciating how we intellectually structure and relate; recognising social rules and roles; informing others; prescribing; reflecting in a critical way; defining the purpose and task; co-creating a safe learning environment; meeting relational and dialogical needs.

Reflecting upon Emotional-Transferential Phenomenon: *[Expressing and directing emotional energy – developing emotional intelligence]* Learning about our emotional responses and patterns: understanding and expressing feelings; releasing blockages of emotional energy; reviewing how our present relates to our past; raising awareness to family scripts; releasing ourselves from the presenting past.

Reflecting upon Imaginal-Projective Phenomenon: *[Exploring and integrating imagination with the self – developing self intelligence]* Surfacing the hidden self; identifying sub-personalities; illuminating inner motives and ego defences; unpacking how imagination informs us; exploring our persona and ego needs; undoing projective identifications and control dramas; raising the shadow.

Reflecting upon Intuitive-Transpersonal Phenomenon: *[Becoming and speculating upon potential beyond the self – developing spiritual intelligence]* Exploring where we truly belong; valuing ourselves and others; becoming authentic; developing holistic vision; illuminating life's purpose; awakening to wisdom above and beyond the self; relating ourselves to the cosmos (after Barber 2012).

The transpersonal/intuitive level was found to underpin them all.

I sometimes attune to the above orientations to better illuminate where I am standing 'holistically' right now, i.e.:

(Reflecting on Physical/Sensory Phenomena – Life as Sensed) I sit ten floors up on the terrace amongst the roof garden. I notice the damp perfume of rain upon leaves, a slight warm breeze caresses my face. A drowsiness descends as I close my eyes to better contact my body. I breathe through my diaphragm to ground myself energetically in the moment. I feel energised. Opening eyes colours seem brighter, I feel physically present and eager to move. I rise and walk to a garden table. The initial page of this chapter flaps before me in the breeze.

(Reflecting on Socio-Cultural Phenomena – Life as Taught) I remember this terrace before we brought in trees, its clinical barrenness. A visual picture surfaces from memory and I find myself comparing this to now. I begin to wonder what our neighbours think of the garden and us. Do they see us as eccentric or a little mad? We are noticeably different after all, a young Romanian wife with an old Brit! We press all the stereotypes!

(Reflecting on Emotional-Transferential Phenomena – Life as Felt) That last reflection leaves me uncomfortable, feeling isolated and fearing misunderstood. As if on trial. Shades of paranoia born of being in a strange land and alien no doubt. I laugh at myself. Never too late to be caught by old stuff, relishing difference yet wanting to belong.

(Reflecting on Imaginal-Projected Phenomena – Life as Imagined) I notice I am deeper into imagined material now, bordering on projection. It's true I'm still unconventional, but hopefully not rebellious. I no longer need to feel special these days to compensate for my sense of being rejected and unloved. I have ceased to be the over-achiever, but then again, why am I writing this Chapter? I haven't written for some years, what am I putting to rest?

(Reflecting on Intuitive-Transpersonal Phenomena – Life as Guided) Relaxing I let go my thought and imagination. Breathing to my heart I settle into silence. I repeat: 'What am I putting to rest?' A host of contenders arise: times of professional solidarity when I chose to hold my tongue than speak my truth and cause offence to colleagues; playing the professional game in private practice. As to the major celebration – more recently freeing myself and my Gestalt from public service. Is this chapter a rite-of-passage – from professionalised Gestalt to individuated Gestalt? I guess this will infuse my narrate.

It is at the transpersonal level we synthesise the whole to distil authentic meaning. Other levels merely supply data.

Though it may appear a 'no brainer', especially to a Gestalt audience, to raise awareness than to blindly act-out, most prefer to remain confined by physical reality comforted by 'life as it is socially taught to be'! Gestalt is up-tight and personal! Why cut through the crap to step into the unknown? Why set all the creatures of our psychic swamp free? Better a peaceful life? Not surprisingly a 'surrender to common ignorance' is all too rife. But beware, take risks and your personal psychological territory grows, play safe and it shrinks!

Gestalt – Humanism in Action?

Over the years, I found that whether a person stayed stuck or met his creative challenges depended on the degree of Humanism that informed our work. It set conditions which increased our ability to engage intuitive-transpersonal exploration.

Let's remind ourselves of how humanistic beliefs and principles pan-out to generate a transpersonal notion of 'social health':

Holism suggests that a person's mental, physical, intellectual, emotional and spiritual qualities are integral to `everything they do' and `all they are'. Consequently, an individual is best approached as a whole mind-body-spiritual being rather than reduced to one or more of their parts. As every thing is multi-faceted and multi-influenced, we are cautioned that there are no easy answers or simple solutions to human problems. *I approach individuals, groups and organisations as organic entities, which, composed of conscious and unconscious elements form a 'living experiential field', in which they are embedded, influence, and in turn influenced by.*

Autonomy supports the notion that given opportunity and resources individuals are best placed to diagnose and resolve their own problems, for they know more about themselves than I or anyone else will ever do. *I watch and listen very carefully to what groups and individuals present, follow what emerges, share personal observations while inquiring into dynamics we co-create. In this way I act as a flexible resource who helps others contact their own inner wisdom.*

Experiential inquiry encourages us to meet life in an open inquiring way, to attend to the unique nature of present relationships and to experiment with owning the whole of ourselves. *I encourage people to take nothing for granted and to question everything. Through a focus upon `what is unique' and ongoing examination of our perceptions, beliefs and relationships, I seek to illuminate awareness in a living experiential cooperative inquiry.*

Democracy supports the notion that we are interdependent rather than independent, and suggests that reason and negotiation should inform all our decision-making. In this vein transparency rather than authoritative imposition and covert agendas inform our social actions. *Holding this in mind I negotiate a client-centred menu where everyone is involved in forming the `how' and `what' of what's on offer. Democracy also keeps me alert to the need for healthy "I – Thou" relationships and keeps me watchful of communication that slides towards an ego-centric "I – I" or a reductionist "I – It" stance to life, self or others.*

Lose sight of the above principles and I suggest you lose touch with Gestalt's dialogical and ethical base, its relational art.

Humanistic psychology rebuffs scientific approaches to psychology, which it deems dehumanising and incapable of capturing the richness of human consciousness. Its influence has sadly waned in most modern Gestalt trainings. Lip-service is paid right enough, but the cut-and-thrust of an open humanistic group devoted to self-actualisation has all but gone.

So what greater purpose does working in a Humanistic way serve? Well, it paves a route to super- health, namely 'self actualisation', which encapsulates an aptitude towards: perceiving reality efficiently; tolerating uncertainty; accepting ourselves and others for what they are; spontaneity in thought and behaviour; maintaining a good sense of humour; being problem-centred rather than self-centred; high creativity; staying resistive to en-culturalistion but not purposely unconventional; demonstrative of concern for the welfare of mankind while deeply appreciative of the basic experiences of life in a child-like way; establishing deep satisfying relationships with a few rather than court the friendship of many; looking at life philosophically and objectively (Maslow 1965). This is the 'super-health' to which I aspire and seek to advance. From where it's a short step to the transpersonal.

Currently, in the UK, Gestalt is more often formally taught than experientially lived. In consequence too many Gestaltists end-up non-actualised. I was lucky enough to experience a humanistic group-centred training in the 70s and early 80s. Later, when professional accreditation kicked in, caught by a desire to be successful, professionally, I sold out and sampled institutional Gestalt. In role as a Gestalt Psychotherapists, do we go with tradition or confront it? Do we succumb to being a paid-up members of the concrete jungle and nod through I-It relationships as the norm? Hopefully not. But can a robust humanistic culture survive unscathed in our reductionist society?

Gestalt – Drowning in Professional Confluence?

I do not decry the value of Gestalt Psychotherapy, yet must nevertheless voice fears that Professionalization has turned it into a safe social animal with over-formalized training respectful if far too many unhealthy cultural introjects. Why do we court 'evidence based practice' which venerates quantitative rather than qualitative data? Or champion the medicalization of DSM (diagnostic and statistical manual) diagnosis? Must we become sentinels of mental health policing out the insane cum unadapted? And who is to say society is a reliable judge of mental health? Not I, for I ascribe to the notion that we live in a sick society that is in danger of getting increasingly sicker! If I am right and society is sick, then health must surely exist in the countercultural domain!

What would Fritz Perl's make of post-modern Gestalt and our drive to sit amongst 'the great and the good'? Look at how many distance ourselves from Fritz. Laura Perls was more user-friendly. Carl Rogers said of the Perls, if they come from Laura – open the doors they are just like us, person-centered, but if they come from Fritz – close the door firmly! (Zinker in conversation with the author). How many of us have raged against Fritz, attacked him for his inappropriateness and chosen the safer path of a watered-down mother-friendly Gestalt in keeping with 'the Nanny State'? Too bloody many I propose. Bloody-mindedness and confrontation can be a powerful therapeutic tools. And 'males' aren't always bad guys.

Has there been a more ruthlessly authentic autobiographical account than Fritz's autobiography – 'In and Out of the Garbage Pail'? (Perls

1972). How many master practitioners would dare share their masturbation and madness with a listening audience? But this not what we encourage our clients to do? I would much prefer a Gestaltist like Fritz who scares me awake than one that lulls me to sleep, yet the latter seem to be emerging from Gestalt training at a rate of knots. How can sleep walkers wake other sleep walkers?

So what has 'really informed' my Gestalt? Not so much my training, as times spent walking towards my fears while remaining true to my heart – life! For instance, pre-training preparing my psychic ground by escaping a controlling and hyper-critical mother by going to Art College rather than taking the safe job she was nagging me to do; after Art College purging my over-protective childhood working as a deckhand and earning my spurs as a working-man in rough-and-tumble with other men. Then Gestalt therapy came into my life to support my coming through major surgery with new learning born of vulnerability; sitting with my son by his deathbed while honouring his contract that I wouldn't grieve in his presence but stay true to the healthy humorous here-and-now relationship we had always enjoyed in our life together; remaining with a dementing partner as Alzheimer's forced her to no longer recognize me or know her self; daring to marry a woman 36 years my junior; siring a daughter and moving to Romania in my late sixties. Gestalt raised these latter incidents to soul work, and life in turn crafted my Gestalt by deepening my presence. Without being bruised by life, what price empathy, let alone appreciation of a reality over and above the self?

At the last, authentic present-time-awareness is born of ego-surrender and dissolution of the need to impress or gain ascendance over others. Enlightenment and wholeness are kissing-cousins. Hindrances to enlightenment have counterparts in Gestalt notions of 'blocks to contact', projection and introjection, which we dissipate to reach the transcendence of 'the-here-and-now'. Indeed, what is not transcendent is not Gestalt!

Gestalt, akin to other spiritual traditions, encourages us to empty our mind, to 'lose our heads and come to our senses'. So that with an open mind and heart we might be guided by what is vibrant, alive and unfolding. If you can't do this you haven't got Gestalt. For like Zen, Gestalt rips the conventional World apart to encourage something other to burst in. In this light, Gestalt education is less like filling a bucket than lighting a fire.

As psychotherapy increasingly quenches its thirst for social acceptance, gains respectability and grows ever more 'professional,' it becomes increasingly difficult for it to challenge, let alone cure social dis-at-ease, for it becomes part of the problem.

Psychotherapy, standing amongst other organs of the State, Education, Religion and Medicine in the shape of Medical Psychiatry, becomes another tool of socially imposed intra-psychic self- discipline. What is the consulting room but a culturally instituted confessional, where psychotherapists act as educators, psychological guides and father confessors all rolled into one? Hereby we become doctors of the psychological interior employed to perform inter-psychic surgery in the interests of purging the community of critical thought? I am not the first to recognize this (Laing 1985; Masson 1988; Isack, & Hook 1995). When you become a signatory of society you sanctify rather than rectify social control (Hurvitz 1974). Working within a conventionally exploitative money-exchanging commercial relationship also recreates self-ostracizing and pathologizing elements, conditions that bring clients to us in the first place. How healthy is this?

When awareness is full and steady our habitual resistances cease to interrupt moment-to-moment contact and we see ourselves and our lives with clarity – becoming available for others. Suspending labelling and meaning-making allows us to rely on insight and intuition rather than analysis. Hereby insight emerges in the moment from the moment. This process is intimately penetrating and deeply cleansing – and all we have to do is invite it in.

Gestalt, building on the premise that perception is more than a sum of the parts, through enhanced awareness and concentrated 'connectedness' opens a portal to an 'Eternal Thou' (Hycner 1993). It reminds us we live in an intelligent self-organising universe. Quantum physics tells us that vibrating fields of energy are much more fundamental than matter, that there are 'no things' to study only vibrating relationships, that the solidity of matter is dependent on the vibration of molecules and awareness itself changes molecular vibration (Schwartz et al 2005).

Gestalt – Ways to Freedom?

So what are we to do? Well, we need to 'be' Gestalt rather than 'do' Gestalt. To divorce ourselves from over-professionalisation; transfuse a heady dose of Humanism and humanistic inquiry into our work; honour transcendent aspects of the human condition and be guided by moment to moment awareness; foster self-actualisation; last but not

CHAPTER 3: GESTALT AS A LIVING SPIRITUAL PRACTICE?

least we need to live through and invite others into moments of impasse. And until we are strong enough to live beyond it, hold our professionalism ever so lightly without undue reference to society's norms and definitions of health.

So rarely do I hear Gestaltists talking of the impasse these days. Have we become trainers rather than inspired guides? Let's remind ourselves of what the 'impasse' involves. Frustrating a person or group to the degree they feel impaled upon the horns of a psychic dilemma, keeping them there, suspended, between impulse and resistance to arouse what Zen calls 'the Great Doubt' (Berlinger et al 2000). When writing I try to cultivate a similar process, questioning and pushing theory to the point it brainstorms and intellect implodes – am I succeeding with you dear reader? During impasse, the mind enters a state where all alternatives to action and thought are blocked, and intellect, the custodian of our 'taught socialised reality' is finally rendered speechless. This was likened by Perls to anti-existence, a transpersonal meeting where nothingness and emptiness are heightened to a degree we become stuck in the throes of our own phobic avoidance (Perls 1972). At this point, when the mind is like 'a mosquito trying to bite an iron bull', magic begins! Staying aware in the midst of this can liberate an awareness free of self-doubt and contradiction – Satori! (Just et al 2000). Tough love at its best!

Experiencing the impasse is far more important than speculating on field theory, narrating blocks to contact, memorising the DSM or other theoretical introjects. Post impasse there is no going back.

Gestalt doesn't ask us to believe anything, just 'do it to find out'. It is a practical experiential route to enlightenment. Remember, fear is merely a fantasy, something we put between where we are now and where we imagine we could end-up! It is not a real 3-dimensional thing, just unbridled emotion making a drama out of a projected crisis. And the steps to illumination? Put crudely: 'shut up', 'attend' and 'pay attention'. For when we stop our internal chatter, live in the present and focus on what's unfolding, we experience our 'being' as a meaningful part of the Universe. Any Gestaltist worth their salt knows that man and the Universe are not separate but one.

If there's no Zen in your Gestalt there's no bite.

We must attend to the moment, cultivate razor sharp awareness and go all the way into 'the experiential now' – if we are to facilitate others to do the same. Remember, Gestalt is not a method but 'a way of being'. Let's not court respectability for the sake of belonging, but stay edgy and counterculture so as to cherish health for the hell of it. Let's wake ourselves up from our sleepy professionally induced respectability to become a force for self-actualisation, the divine and super- health once again.

> Truly 'be' with your clients, share your humanity, breathe them in, share your observations and intuitions – gently grow their 'Great Doubt'.

So I've shared my dream, a Gestalt preparation wherein a self-actualised transpersonal presence is cultivated and an Encounter Group is facilitated on humanistic lines serving a process-led experiential curriculum. Institutionalised tuition with formal examinations quantitatively assessed, where academic papers and case studies are read and produced stimulates old paradigm thinking to hold sway, displacing process-alive Gestalt. To be accepted by academia and accredited, the hoops we jump through induce us to 'throw out our Gestalt baby with the bathwater'. In this way we sell-out the qualitative richness and compromise the humanistic ethics of our paradigm. Far better we expose ourselves and trainees to shamanistic workshops where we might develop an ability to 'feel the field' rather than theorise about it.

So here is the problem – now craft your own solution.

Take out the developmental thrust towards self-actualisation and things transpersonal, ruthless authenticity over-and-above societal expectations, education of the intuition, humanism plus the impasse, and you soil Gestalt's unique Zen-like core. Better you do Gestalt beyond the social pail, in fact don't even call it Gestalt nor anything else or society will ostracise or professionally sanitise you. Just live it as a spiritual way!

Am I inciting you to become outlaws? To fly under society's radar as travelling healers? Perhaps even to be Gestalt Shamans!

References

Barber, P. (2012). *Facilitating Change in Groups & Teams: A Gestalt Approach to Mindfulness*. Faringdon: Libri Publishing.

Hurvitz, N. (1974). 'Psychotherapy as a means of social control'. *Journal of Consulting and Clinical Psychology, (40)*2, pp. 232-239.

Isack, S. and Hook, D. (1995). 'The psychological imperialism of psychotherapy', University of Witwatersrand, 20 October. Witwatersrand, South Africa: 1st Annual Qualitative Methods Conference.

Just, B., Feldhaus, B. and Bearinger, O. (2000). Impasse. *Gestalt!* (5)2, Early Fall.

Laing, R. (1985). *Wisdom, madness and folly: The making of a psychiatrist 1927-1957.* London: Macmillan.

Maslow, A. (1965). 'Cognition of Being in Peak Experience.' *Journal of Genetic Psychology,* (94) pp. 43-66.

Masson, J. (1988). *Against therapy: Emotional tyranny and the myth of psychological healing.* New York: Atheneum.

Perls, F. (1972) *In and Out the Garbage Pail.* New York: Bantam Books.

Schwartz, J., Stapp, H. and Beauregard, M. (2005). 'Quantum Physics in Neuroscience and Psychology: A Neurophysical Model of Mind-Brain Interaction'. *Philosophical Transactions of the Royal Society of London. Series B, Biological Sciences.* 360(1458), pp. 1309-27.

Szasz, T. (1979) *The myth of psychotherapy: mental healing as religion, rhetoric, and repression.* Oxford: Oxford University Press.

Wheway, K. (1999). Spirituality and Selfhood. *British Gestalt Journal,* (8)2, pp. 118-29.

Zinker, J. (2001) 'The Present Isn't What it Used to Be: A Gestalt Encounter with Joseph Zinker, an interview by Paul Barber', *British Gestalt Journal,* (10)1, pp. 29-37.

II. THE GESTALT PRACTITIONER

Chapter 4: A Short Note on the "Use of Self" and Gestalt

Mee-Yan Cheung-Judge

There has long been a gentle debate among Gestalt and OD practitioners as to where the concept of Use of Self (UoS) originated. This chapter aims to (I) look at where this concept came from and explore the background that gave rise to the concept; (II) review the definitions of UoS; (III) briefly revisit the concept of the field – the relational ground for UoS; and (IV) end with some practice implications for practitioners.

I. The Origin of "Use of Self" – History of Gestalt psychology and Gestalt psychotherapy

One could not do justice to the origin of the concept of UoS without going back to the field and theories of Gestalt psychology and Gestalt therapy. Both fields germinated in Europe. By tracing the flow of their historical context, the birth of the concept will become clearer.

A. Gestalt Psychology

In the late 1800s, two publications helped to give legitimacy and validity to psychology as an investigative science. The first was by Wilhelm Wundt, *The Principles of Physiological Psychology* (1874), which introduced the rigors of scientific inquiry and put psychology on the map of investigative science, especially the investigation of the conscious processes. The second publication was Franz Brentano's *Psychology from an Empirical Standpoint* (1874). He had built his work on scientific methods backed up by a strong philosophical root. He and his student, Christian von Ehrenfels, developed a general theory of complex perception, emphasizing the possibility of unbiased description of inner experience as the basis of scientific inquiry. Sixteen years later (1890), Christian von Ehrenfels published *On Gestalt Quality*, coining the term *Gestalt* from his and Brentano's work on perception. Many believe this was when the Gestalt School of Psychology was born.

The Berlin School of Gestalt Psychology played a critical role to advance the field. The work of four people: Max Wertheimer, Kurt Koffka, Wolfgang Kohler, and Kurt Lewin became the bedrock of the School, especially the work of Wertheimer on perceptual grouping and perception of movement. They, together with others, e.g. Goldstein, Fritz Perls and Lore Posner (Laura Perls) played critical roles in reinforcing the scientific approach to psychology while laying the path for Gestalt therapy. Goldstein asserted that Gestalt perceptual psychology could be applied to the entire human condition, and that philosophy has a legitimate place in medicine.

Laura Perls studied Husserl's (a student of Brentano) work on Phenomenological Reduction with Paul Tillich, and later with Martin Buber. She and Fritz Perls, under the guidance of Goldstein, were exposed to a breadth of philosophical heritage through Tillich, Kierkegaard, Heidegger, Husserl, and Scheler. Lewin developed field theory, action research, and system dynamics, etc. They all played parts in laying the foundational platform for the study of SELF. The excitement during that period came from the realisation that when psychology is sustained by its philosophical roots and scientific methods, an existentially and phenomenologically based *psychotherapy* can be made possible.

What is Gestalt psychology? One of the original writers described it thus: "a thing given in perception as the Gestalt quality of a sum of perceived characters" (Meinong 1909 quoted by Mulligan and Smith 1988:129) – which literally means the "whole is greater than the sum of its parts." Put in another way, Gestalt psychology is the study of perception and behaviour from the standpoint of an individual's response to configurational wholes rather than by analysing their constituents.

B. Gestalt Therapy

Gestalt therapy became a dominant school of thinking as a result of an intended departure by a group of philosophers, psychoanalysts, and scientists from the 19th century medical view of psychoanalysis, of which Freud was the main proponent. While Freud acknowledged the impact a repressive and conservative Victorian Society could have on a person's "disease", his model was a medical one and his classifications of id, ego, superego were part of his belief in psychoanalytic dissection. Freud's advice to young psychoanalysts confirmed this (Stepansky 1999):

> *"I cannot advise my colleagues too urgently to model themselves during psychoanalytic treatment on the superego,*

who puts aside all his feelings, even his human sympathy, and concentrates his mental forces on the single aim of performing the operation as skilfully as possible."

Contrary to the belief that Fritz Perls was the father of Gestalt Therapy, Bowman and Nevis (2005), named the contribution of others who joined forces to question the work of Freud. They included:
- **Rank** explored the role of the "here and now" in the psychoanalytic setting
- **Adler** examined the role of paradox in therapy
- **Federn** developed preliminary concepts around ego boundaries
- **Ferenzi** championed the active involvement of the analyst and emphasized the subject nature of interpretation
- **Reich** emphasized the concept of "organismic self-regulation" and his general theory of "character armor"
- **Goodman** was credited with writing most of the theoretical material of Gestalt therapy with Fritz Perls
- **Laura Perls** upheld the philosophical and aesthetic vs technical root of Gestalt therapy. She believed it is the existential-phenomenological approach that allows an experiential and experimental methodology in Gestalt Therapy.

The above group saw Gestalt therapy as a possible engine to counteract the destructive world view at that time: where diversity was persecuted, where linear causality toward any paradigm was hailed, where atomic focus overrode a holistic model of existence, where individualistic survival took precedence over relational connectedness in life. They believed that through the confluence of the diversity of its contributors and their personal beliefs and values, e.g. Hasidism, Taoism, physics, feminism, radical individualism, relational psychology, the possibility of a better world could be demonstrated.

Bowman gave a working definition of Gestalt therapy (1998:106):

> *"Gestalt therapy is a process psychotherapy with the goal of improving one's contact in community and with the environment in general. This goal is accomplished through aware, spontaneous and authentic dialogue between client and therapist. Awareness of differences and similarities is encouraged while interruptions to contact are explored in the present therapeutic relationship."*

It is worth noting the movement from Gestalt psychology to Gestalt therapy reflects the developmental split between the scientists and the practitioners – the latter believe the world can be changed, while the former wanted to continue the rigorous pursuit of scientific inquiry. They were called the "Gestalt-oriented scientists".

In 1951, Fritz Perls, Hefferline, and Goodman coined the name in *Gestalt therapy: Excitement and Growth in the Human Psychology*. Together they also gave birth to the New York Institute for Gestalt Therapy – the first professional training group.

During this period, Kurt Lewin's work on action research, systems dynamics and especially field theory, together with Goldstein's field ideas gained wide recognition that virtually all fields are open for investigation.

C. Central tenets of Gestalt Therapy – the foundational platform for Use of Self

As more publications appeared and more training schools and institutes were established, the central tenets of Gestalt therapy began to emerge with clarity from its richly historical, philosophical and scientific setting. Some of the following points can be attributed to specific individuals while others come from composite writings:

- Goldstein's concept of the *organism as a whole* and the ability of the human organism in adapting to the environment, especially in adversity – not how one system does something to another, but how systems mutually act and react to each other (a shift from Freud's mechanistic conception of human nature to a more dynamic and positive approach to life).
- Lewin's work on the *inseparability of the organism in the environment* and the *field perspectives*. For a Gestalt therapist, the field is the personal perception of one's environment, not merely a subjective reality but a relational product that is centred on the contact boundary between the internal and external – how the self's experiences and needs interact with the environment's demands or conditions. In that sense, *the field* is a process not a system.
- Fritz Perls' Cycle of Experience which gives the centrality of Gestalt practice (both consulting and therapeutic work) in addressing interruptions to full and meaningful completion of the COE.
- According to Judith Brown, Martin Buber's exposition of *presence* and *mutuality*, and his philosophy and values of

presence, authenticity, dialogue and inclusion, (*I and Thou* publication 1923/1958), have become the "goal of every intervention in Gestalt therapy" (1980:55). She cited Buber's work as the most important influence on Gestalt therapy in terms of its therapeutic values.
- The Reichian concept of *organisimic self-regulation* shaped the function of psychotherapy, as human nature is capable of self-regulation. When an organism makes contact with the environment, change occurs.
- Kierkegaard's belief that *truth is subjective* – passionate choices, strong convictions, and personal experience compose an individual's truth. All observation is a phenomenological viewpoint from a place, time and perspective, hence multiple vs knowable "objective" realities exist.
- Heidegger's belief in *"being"* as more fundamental than consciousness.
- Husserl's belief that investigative work should be through the *phenomenological method*.
- Edgar Rubin (Rubin's Vase) identified the figure-ground concept in his 1915 doctoral thesis "Synsoplevede Figurer." Subsequently Friedlaender's theory of *figure and ground formulations* of the Gestalt theory, together with his concept of the *"fertile void"* helped us to understand the emergent Gestalt. His philosophy of *"creative indifference"* also shaped the role of the therapists. His philosophical contribution led to a method of integrating polarities.
- Goodman's immersion in Eastern philosophical literature directed the Gestalt therapist not just to change psychoanalysis for individuals, but to *change society* as he believed that a healthier individual would produce a healthier society.
- The shared world view of "weltanschauung" or *holism tendency* (vs atomism) as fundamental in nature. "Lives and collective systems intertwine and need to be considered together as a unified field" (Parlett 1997:16). This led to the methodology that causality cannot be found out through atomistic investigation even though it can reveal correlation.
- *Awareness* is critical to support organism self-regulation. Through one's sensory, affective and cognition awareness, one can make intentional choices to enable change to happen. As a *self-process,* awareness happens when "self" interacts with the other, and the environment. The original meaning of awareness is a "glowing light" inside the self, serving as an inner witness of

the thinking, feeling, and observing by the SELF in the here and now. It is a critical meaning-making process.
- *Meaning making is a crucial process* for therapists to help patients/clients to increase their awareness of the figures and ground process. A "figure" stands out from the background as what is salient to clients and us. Once an individual has feelings about the figure and ground configuration, then the meaning-making process is happening.

What are the practice implications from such central tenets? It is permissible for the therapists/consultants/helpers to pay attention not only to what is figural for the client, but also for themselves. It is their experiences, observations and the use of their whole self (not just tools and techniques, or pre-determined methodology) as creative instruments that will create a different presence (relational presence), an optimal condition for the client to do their own work towards wholeness. This is articulated clearly by Perls (1969) who believed Freud's approach to have the therapist half-hidden in the wings would encourage regression and transference on the part of the patient, hence it is important to bring the therapist and patient together onto the centre stage to illuminate the relationship as clearly as possible. This was also pointed out by Rainey and Jones (2014, p.106) "....the concept of UoS whereby the consultant is granted permission to use personal experience in service of the goals of the clients".

From the Gestalt beliefs, the concept of UoS can be summed up in the following ways : a) we will need to bring our whole self to work with our clients; b) who we are and how we continue to evolve are fundamental resources in our work with people; c) the intentionality we have to create collective good for the systems we work with will guide how we choose what to do and how to maintain flexibility in action; d) the reverse learning and growth from partnership with our clients will further deepen our awareness of who we are, who others are, and generally how to develop our instrumentality.

II. Definitions of Use of Self

There are many definitions of UoS in literature. Some stem from Gestalt and others come from disciplines like social work, anthropology, coaching, other psychotherapeutic schools, and OD. For now, we will mainly look at the Gestalt and OD writers' definition.
- "The use of self is the way in which one acts upon one's

observations, values, feelings and so forth, in order to have an effect on the other." Nevis (1987:125) He also expanded the use of self as happening when we allow our own sensations, feelings, and knowing to inform and support richer and potentially more insightful intervention into client's system.
- "The OD practitioner is not only to stand for and express certain values, attitudes, and skills, but to use these in a way to stimulate, and perhaps evoke from the client, actions necessary for movement on its problems...the aim is to take advantage of the issues of differences, marginality, and attraction by the client so as to use oneself in the most powerful way." Nevis (1987:54)
- "The development of the self as instrument is a continuous process of learning about one's conscious and unconscious reactions in different settings with different people." Berg (1990)
- "Use of self is acting on feelings, observations, and thoughts to advance the work of the client." Rainey and Jones (2014:107)
- "Use of self is the process of acting upon a complex set of factors related to the consultant, client, and the practice of OD. It requires attending to self and client while honouring the values that are fundamental to OD… UoS is the integration of consultant (values, assumptions, beliefs, biases, tendencies), client (attending and engaging with integrity and purposeful intention) and OD (values, principles, theory, practices)." Rainey and Jones (2014:114)
- "Use of self is the conscious use of one's whole being in the intentional execution of one's roles for effectiveness in whatever the current situation is presenting. The purpose is to be able to execute a role effectively, for others and the system they're in, without personal interference (e.g. bias, blindness, avoidance, and agendas) …to have clear intention and choice." Jamison, Auron and Shechtman (2010).
- "To be able to be relevant in the here and now takes a person who is centred, sensitive, flexible who has tolerance for ambiguity and who can stay with the immediate situation and help those with whom s/he is working to flow once again with the river." Tannenbaum (1997:173)
- "The simplest way we know to talk about Use of Self is to link the concepts of self-awareness, perceptions, choices and actions as the fundamental building blocks of our capacities to be effective agents of the change. Hopefully to make a better world and to develop our own potential for doing so to the

fullest in the processes." Seashore, Shawver, Thompson and Mattare (2004:42)
- "Use of self consists of intentional, conscious and deliberate choices which result in action/behaviours taken to bring about change." Seashore, Shawver, Thompson and Mattare (2004:44)
- Energetic availability: Fluid responsibility. Chidias, (2018).
- Self-Efficacy and Self Agency. Bandura, (1997).
- Presence. Buber (1923).

Two things are noticeable from the above definitions:
(1) the practitioner's UoS takes place within a "field" (a critical theoretical lens of Gestalt), sometimes referred to as a "relational field" or "unitary field". Regardless of the precise name, they all point to the fact that all things are interconnected, and where self and others are constantly making contact in a mutuality and inclusive manner to shape and reshape the evolution of self.
(2) Buber's term "presence", has been upheld as an interchangeable term with UoS. What is presence? According to Nevis (1987), Rainey Tolbert and Hanafin (2006) and Rainey and Jones (2014), presence emerges from and is experienced as the distinctive integration of the whole of who and what the practitioner is – affection, perception, cognition, behaviour – that is interesting enough to achieve and maintain a learning and development partnership with the client. These writers believe that presence is the mix of essence of the whole self and awareness with intent and impact. Just like the use of self, presence is a relational process and can be cultivated, because it takes place in the context of relationship and connection. In fact, Chidiac (2018: 47) said "presence can be positioned at the heart of the Gestalt approach because it is a core condition for the effective instrumentality of the practitioners, which in Gestalt is called the Use of Self." Presence is the epitome of the use of self.

III. The Concept of the "Field" – the relational ground for UoS

All relationships take place within a field which can be a specific "here and now" temporal situation or can be a bigger and longer-term macro field. Even though it is hard to define, Malcolm Parlett (2005: 43) said

CHAPTER 4: A SHORT NOTE ON THE "USE OF SELF" AND GESTALT

"the concept of the field has become both indispensable and theoretically central." He went on to say that Field theory, the field perspective, the relational field or the field paradigm are central to Gestalt.

The question is when the UoS requires us to make a holistic decision on what to do, which lenses will help us gain a fuller and more integrated understanding of people's experiences and behaviour? Perl et al (1994:4) stated that "In any psychological investigation whatever, we must start from the interacting of the organism and its environment...Let us call this interacting of organism and environment in any function the "organism/environment field." According to him, this "founding orientation" is different from most psychological theories where emphasis is put on investigating individual ego states, personality, psychological tendencies, and their motivation to self-actualisation. These parts will only offer so much understanding of the person's behaviour, because human behaviour can never be explained in isolation from its natural settings. In fact, the danger in focusing mainly on the individual's intra psychic psychological processes is that we will lose what Gestalt theorists call the holistic stance, without which a fuller, more integrated understanding of people's experience will be hard to grasp. This means in understanding of one but not the other (concept of Use of Self and concept of the "field"), our lenses will become myopic and constricted, which will reflect on our practice.

This relational field was captured in an accessible way in 2013 by two UK-based Gestalt writers (Denham Vaughan and Chidiac) in a model calls SOS – **S**elf, **O**ther, and **S**ituation. See Figure 1.

Figure 1 : The SOS (self, other situation) Model Chidiac 2018

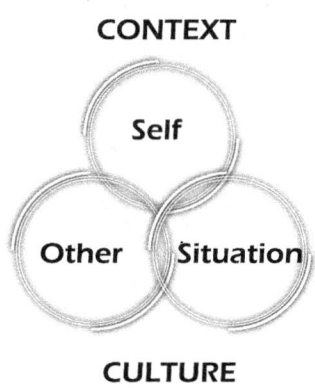

The model "proposes that a relational stance is one that finds a balance between the three interrelated elements
- ***Self*** *– can be seen as either the individual, group, community or organisation.*
- ***Other*** *– is the "other" in the relationship at any given moment. When self-reflecting, this can be the "other within the self", or for a business this can be competitors or allies from whom they differentiate.*
- ***Situation*** *– is the particular set of happenings occurring in any given moment.*

These three do not sit in a vacuum but are embedded in a given context and culture." (Chidias 2018:51-52)

Using the structure of the SOS model, I expanded it to give a fuller description of the Use of Self, as well as looking at the implications of the relational field theory on our practice.

Figure 2: The Use of Self Framework

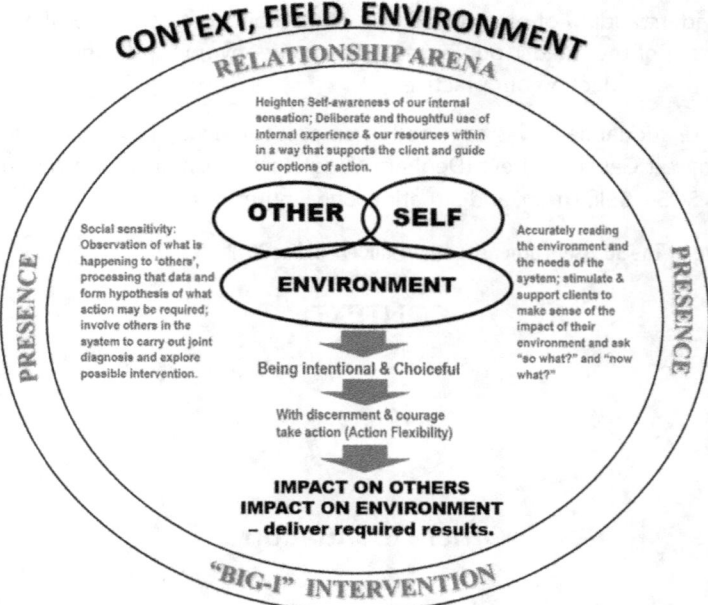

In this model, we start with the three SOS elements within the "field" which Yontef (1993:297) defined as "a totality of mutually influencing forces that together form a unified interactive whole." We (the self), our clients (others), and we together (self and others) are all parts in relation with the larger whole. The intimate interconnectedness between us (the therapist/consultants/helpers) and the many "others" puts us inevitably in position to impact on the "others" as we make contact across boundaries, moment by moment using what we know, what we care about, what we observe, what we feel....to span across boundaries to make things happen. We also develop our ability simultaneously not just to use who we are to support clients in their reality, but to stay open to the data emerging from others to impact on us.

This holistic field perspective enables us to hold all things together in spite of the ongoing chaos. In the "here and now", we need to intervene in the system to accomplish the system-required goals. The intervention requires us to make relationships our top work, to put ourselves on the line, to deepen our self-awareness of what is going on both within us and outside of us. We also need to develop an increasing sense of social sensitivity so that our ability to observe accurately of what is going on will help us to decide what intervention will be necessary. Analysing the relevance of the options of interventions in the context of where we are will require the deployment of our discernment and courage before taking appropriate action. It is then we can say we are using our presence to make the Big I intervention choicefully and intentionally.

Finally, the Gestalt sense of "self" is never static, but fluid in its nature. The belief is that no one needs to be locked into a past narrative and stay there for life. When we use ourselves to impact others and the environment, we ourselves will also be impacted by our contact with our various "others" within "multiple fields."

IV. Some Practice Implications for Practitioners

What are the implications of the expanded model on practitioners? Four areas to consider:
1. Be diligent to know the complex context we work in – political, social, psychological, physical, spiritual, cultural, time orientation, psychoanalytical, psychodynamic world, etc. Within the complex context, the practitioners need to work with many "others" within a relational arena, across a living system where divergence is inherent, yet holism is the only perspective for us

to use in the work. When different "others" will need different support because the environment will have different impacts on them, we need to realistically accept that while some formulaic guides for practitioners can be helpful, ultimately the real test for practitioners is 1) our ability to identify what emerges from the "here and now" as our and "others'" boundaries get in contact and disrupted; 2) our willingness and ability to do "real time calibration and re-design" based on our sense of judgement; 3) our presence, our phenomenological inquiry, and our dialogical approach.

2. Second, in this field approach, there is no right or wrong way to intervene. This is not saying any intervention will do. But it is saying intervention within a fundamental relational stance should emphasize the mutuality of co-creating, co-designing, sharing and making meaning, gaining understanding of mutual reality of what the shared field is – through data gained from phenomenological inquiry, and better intervention will be a natural outcome. This approach will require putting ourselves into the others' perspective, feeling what they feel without giving up our own sense of self. Accepting the person, confirming our sense of their existence and future potential, while staying authentic with ourselves is what Gestalt practitioners call practicing the "inclusion and confirmation" spirit. In that way, we help to create what Lewin called the "life space" for contact. In that context, growth and change will happen as Carl Hodges (1997) said "contact organises the field".

3. Third, in any situation, it is crucial that we practice the art of observing others and the environment, scanning for data all the time, processing it while managing the continuous flood of new external data coming in. The challenge is to continuously hone our social sensitivity while paying attention to our own internal sensations, forming working hypotheses and, discerning moment by moment what needs to happen. When we intervene, action flexibility will be required as the "here and now", while anticipating boundary disruption will produce unpredictable consequences. We also need to perfect "in the moment" deployment of our own precious resources to intervene with the dynamic system to achieve results. Through our own observation and mutual feedback with "others", we develop action flexibility to act based on the emerging data.

4. Finally, we need to continue to develop a heightened sense of self-awareness and an ability to process what we have seen,

heard, and experienced between those contact boundaries. We need to see our "selves" in action to create the desired impact within the relationship arena. With feedback from others, we learn the value of our presence in holding, reassuring, guiding the process of work (or not). As we become more confident in expanding our cognitive power, our heart work, experimenting with how to become a more courageous intervener, we will witness the potency of our SELF-which is our Big I in action. Our ability to do so will also depend heavily on the frequency and type of self-care habits we have. Like a car, we will need refuelling and servicing regularly. The more integrated we become in using our presence to hold, challenge, and develop the system, the greater ease we will have in using ourselves in the moment to make the "Big I intervention."

One of the practices and developmental challenges most of us have in our journey in Use of Self is how we manage the interaction between the three circles of self, others, and environment, and the constant boundary-spanning exchange between them. With experience, developing the ability to balance comfortably on that three-legged stool, especially in the "here and now" moments, will continue to be major life work for most of us.

Summary

This article is intended to, through tracing Gestalt's rich history and its range of definitions, revitalise the concept of UoS. The current times carry many complex factors that have played a role to diminish the confidence of many "system helpers/practitioners". We need to fall back and hold onto what differentiates Gestalt and OD practice from most other branches of consultancy – i.e. our ability to use our "self" in the here and now to work effectively for the clients. We must increase the desirability of our community to those whom we serve. My final exhortation in a "Use of Self" journey is (1) put relationship as our top work; (2) be a holistic and system thinker; (3) deepen our awareness of who we are and our internal workings; (4) determine to use ourselves to serve those systems we work for. Who knows, as those early Gestalt founders thought – through the confluence of our potent use of self, the possibility of a better world can be showcased.

References

Adler, A. (1956). *The Individual Psychology of Alfred Adler* (H. L. Ansbacher and R.R. Ansbacher, Ed. And Trans) New York: Harper and Row.

Bandura, A. (1997). *Self-Efficacy: the Exercise of Control*. W. H. Freeman

Bowman, C. E. (1998). Definitions of Gestalt therapy: Finding Common group. *Gestalt Review*, 2 (2), 97-107.

Bowman, C. E. (2005). The History and Development of Gestalt Therapy (Dialogue Respondent: E. C. Nevis). In Woldt, Ansel L. and Toman, Sarah M. (Ed.). *Gestalt Therapy: History, Theory, and Practice*. London: Sage Publications

Brentano, F. (1999). Psychology from an Empirical Perspective. London: Routledge

Brown, J. (1980). Buber and Gestalt. *Gestalt Journal*, 3 (2), 47-55

Buber, M. (1958). *I and Thou* (R. G. Smith Trans.) New York: Scribner (Original work published 1923)

Burke, W. (1982). *Organisation Development: Principles and Practices*. Boston: Little, Brown and Company.

Chidiac, MA. (2018). *Relational Organisational Gestalt: An Emergent Approach to Organisation Development*. Karnac.

Cheung-Judge, MY. (2012). The Self as an Instrument: A Cornerstone for the Future of OD. *OD Practitioner*, Vol. 44, No 2.

Denham-Vaughan, S. & Chidiac, M-A. (2013). SOS: A relational orientation towards social inclusion. *Mental Health and Social Inclusion*, 17 (2): 100-107

Ehrenfels, C. von. (1988). On Gestalt Qualities. In B. Smith (Ed. & Trans.), *Foundations of Gestalt Theory* (pp. 82-117) Munich: Philosophia (Original work published 1890)

Federn, P. (1952). *Ego Psychology and the Psychoses*. New York: Basic Book.

Friedlaender, S. (2014). His work and influence on Perls was described in *Fritz*, by M. Shepard: Open Book Media.

Funches, D. (1989). The Gifts of the Organisation Development Practitioner. In *The Emerging Practice of Organisation Development* (Ed) by Sikes, W; Drexler, A; Gant, J. Co-published by NTL and University Associates, Inc. CA: San Diego.

Goldstein, K. (1995). *The Organism: A holistic approach to Biology Derived from Pathological Data I Man*. New York: Zone. (Original work published 1939)

Goodman, P. (1997a). The father of the psychoanalytic Movement. In T. Stoehr (Eds) Nature Heals: *The psychological Essays of Paul Goodman*. New York: Free Life Editions (Reprint from Kenyon Review; September 20, 1945)

Goodman, P. (1997b). The Political Meaning of Some Recent Revisions of Freud. In T. Stoehr (Ed.) *Nature Heals: The Psychological Essays of Paul Goodman*. New York: Free Life Editions (Reprinted from Politics, 1945).

Heidegger, M. (1949). The Essence of Truth. In W. Brock (Ed.) *Existence and Being* (R. F. C. Hull and A. Crick, Trans.) New York: Henry Regnery.

Hodges, C. (1997, January). *Field Theory*. Unpublished manuscript presented at New York Institute for Gestalt Therapy.

Husserl, E. (1989). *Ideas Pertaining to a Pure Phenomenology and to a Phenomenological Philosophy – Second Book: Studies in the Phenomenology of Constitution*. (Trans) by R. Rojcewicz and A. Schuwer, Dordrecht: Kluwer.

Husserl, E. (1970). *The Crisis of European Sciences and Transcendental Philosophy*. (Trans) by Carr, D. Evanston: Northwestern University Press. (Original publication 1936/1954)

Jamieson, D.W., Auron, M., Shechtman, D. (2010). Managing Use of Self for Masterful Professional Practice. *OD Practitioner*, Vol.42 No.3.

Kierkegaard, S. (1954). Fear and Trembling and the Sickness unto Death (W. Lowrie, Trans.) Princeton, NJ. Princeton University Press (Original Work published 1941)

Lewin, K. (1938). Will and Need. In W. Ellis (Ed.) *A Source Book of Gestalt Psychology* (pp. 283-299). London: Routledge and Kegan Paul. (Reprinted from *Psychologische Forschung*, 7, 1926)

Lewin, K. (1951). *Field Theory in Social Science: Selected Theoretical Papers*. New York: Harper. 005

Lobb, J. S; Lichtenberg, P. (2005). *Classical Gestalt Therapy Theory*. Sage Book.

McCormick, D., White, J. (2000) Using One's Self as an Instrument for Diagnosis. *Organisation Development Journal*,19 (3).

McLagan, P. (1987). *Models for HRD Practice. American Society for Training and Development*. Va: Alexandria.

Maslow, A. (1968). *Toward a Psychology of Being*. New York: Van Nostrand Reinhold.

Maslow, A. (1971). *The Farther Reaches of Human Nature*. New York: Viking.

Maurer, Rick. (2005). Gestalt Approaches with Organizations and Large Systems. In Woldt, Ansel L. and Toman, Sarah M. (editors) (2005). *Gestalt Therapy: History, Theory, and Practice*. London: Sage Publications

Mulligan, K., & Smith, B. (1988). Mach and Ehrenfels: The Foundations of Gestalt Theory. In B. Smith (Ed.) *Foundations of Gestalt Theory* (pp. 124-157). Munich: Philosophia.

Nevis, E. C. (1987). *Organizational Consulting: A Gestalt Approach*. New York: Gardner.

Nevis, E. C. (Ed.) (1992). *Gestalt Therapy: Perspectives and Applications*. New York: Gardner.

Nevis, E. C. (1997). Gestalt Therapy and Organisation Development: A Historical Perspective, 1930-1996. *Gestalt Review*, 1(2).

Parlett, M. (1991). Reflections on Field Theory. *British Gestalt Journal*, I (2), 69-81.

Parlett, M. (1997). The Unified Field in Practice. *Gestalt Review*, I (1), 10-33.

Parlett, M. (2005). Contemporary Gestalt therapy: Field theory. 10.4135/9781452225661.n3.

Perls, F.S., Hefferline, R., & Goodman, P. (1951). *Gestalt Therapy: Excitement and Growth in the Human Personality*. New York: Julian.

Perls, F.S., Hefferline, R., & Goodman, P. (1994). *Gestalt Therapy: Excitement and Growth in the Human Personality* (revised edition). New York: Julian.

Perls, F. S. (1996a). *Ego, Hunger, and Aggression: The Beginning of Gestalt Therapy*. New York: Random House. (Original work published 1947)

Perls, F. S. (1996b) *Gestalt Therapy Verbatim*. Lafayette, CA: Real People.

Perls, L. (1992). Concepts and Misconceptions of Gestalt Therapy. In E. Smith (Ed.) *Gestalt Voices* (pp. 3-8). Norwood, NJ: Ablex.

Rank, O. (1941). *Beyond Psychology*. Philadelphia, Dover.

Rainey Tolbert, M.A; Hanafin, J. (2006). Use of Self in OD Consulting: What Matters is Presence. In Jones, B. Brazzel, M. (Ed.) *The NTL Handbook of Organisation Development and Change*. San Francisco, CA: Pfeiffer.

Rainey, M. A; Jones, B (2014). Use of Self as an OD Practitioner. In Jones, B. Brazzel, M. (Ed.) *The NTL Handbook of Organisation Development and Change*, Second Edition. San Francisco, CA: Pfeiffer.

Reich, W. (1945). *Character-Analysis*. (T. P. Wolfre, Trans.) New York: Farrar, Straus and Giroux.

Reich, W. (1960). *Wilhelm Reich: Selected Writings* (T. Wolfe, Trans.) New York: Farrar, Straus and Giroux.

Rubin, Edgar (1915), *Synsoplevede Figurer* – PhD thesis, University of Copenhagen.

Seashore, C. N; Shawver, M. N; Thompson, G; Mattare, M. (2004). Doing Good by Knowing Who You Are: The Instrumental Self as an Agent of Change. *OD Practitioner*, Vol. 36, No. 3.

Seashore, C. N; Curran, K.M; Welp, M.G. (1995). *Use of Self as an Instrument of Change*. Presentation paper to 1995 ODN National Conference, Seattle, Washington.

Stephansky, P. (1999). *Freud, Surgery, and the Surgeons*. Hillsdale, NJ: Analytic Press.

Tannenbaum, R. (1997). Of Time and the River, in *Organisation Development Classics*, edited by Van Eynde, Donald F; Hoy Judith C., Van Eynde, Dixie Cody; San Francisco: Jossey-Bass (originally published in *OD Practitioner*, 1979, 11(1)

Tannenbaum, R; Hanna, R. (1985). Holding on, Letting go, Moving on: Understanding a neglected Perspective on Change. In *Human System Development*. Tannenbaum, R; Margullies, N; Massarik, F. (Eds.) San Francisco: Jossey-Bass.

Tschudy, T. (2006). An OD Map: The Essence of Organisation Development. In Jones, B. Brazzel, M. (Ed.) *The NTL Handbook of Organisation Development and Change*. San Francisco, CA: Pfeiffer.

Van Eynde, Donald F; Hoy Judith C., Van Eynde, Dixie Cody; (editors) (1997). *Organisation Development Classics*. San Francisco: Jossey-Bass

Woldt, Ansel L. and Toman, Sarah M. (editors) (2005). *Gestalt Therapy: History, Theory, and Practice*. London: Sage Publications

Wundt, W. (1999). Grundzuge der Physiologischen Psychologie (Principles of Physiological Psychology). In R. Wozniah (Ed.) *Classics in Psychology, 1874 (Vol.10)*. Bristol, UK: Thoemmes. (Original Work published 1874)

Yontef, G. (1993) *Awareness, dialogue and process: Essays on Gestalt Therapy*. Highland, NY: Gestalt Journal Press.

Chapter 5: Four Roles of the Gestalt Intervener: Holistic Presence Using Experiential Learning Theory

Mary Ann Rainey

"Personal feelings and experience are the only realm in which humans are unimpeachable sources of truth." (Buckingham & Goodall, 2019, p.5)

Constant change and complexity are part of the fabric of our lives. Some of us thrive under these circumstances. However, most find it unnerving, disheartening, and at times outright scary. I think of the 21st century as the "age of not knowing" when everyday experiences are so new and unfamiliar that we cannot easily discern what to do or how to do it. Many people expect and respond fairly effectively to small bursts of change. Now they are bombarded by unrelenting disruption and volatility.

Change practitioners – leaders, managers, administrations, consultants, coaches and facilitators – feel the weight of supporting those caught in the throes of this new normal and are seeking additional resources to assist them. If practitioners are to be helpful, they must provide more pragmatic intervention strategies – ones that spark connection, collaboration, and sense of community that effect achievement of desired goas.

One assumption that underpins my work is that unprecedented change requires commitment to continuous learning. Experiential Learning Theory (Kolb, 2015) gives the Gestalt practitioner an additional template for intervening in complex dynamics while keeping continuous learning as the ultimate goal. The framework is the *Four Roles of the Gestalt Intervener* or *FROGI*. It is a coherent and actionable adaptation of Kolb's four modes of learning – concrete experience, reflective observation, abstract conceptualization, and active experimentation – and yields four corresponding ways to intervene:
- *Experiencing,* by attending to *the practitioner's* personal and immediate concrete experience;
- *Noticing,* by observing patterns and themes emerging *from the client and immediate environment;*

- *Grand theorizing,* by making-meaning of what is noticed *from the client and immediate environment* using abstract concept and generalizations;
- *Influencing* the *client's process* and advancing the work through active experimentation.

Experiential Learning Theory is well-suited for the process orientation of Gestalt practice. When the FROGI model is coupled with prevailing Gestalt theory and methods, the practitioner is better prepared to leverage the benefits of change rather than surrender to its burdens. The objective is to forge a more holistic presence – capacity and capability to attend to and respond "on demand" to complex dynamics in a range of ways and at multiple levels of system – individual, two-person, group and larger systems. Holistic presence involves the practitioner's ability to enact all four roles.

To establish context for FROGI, I offer brief backstories of Gestalt practice and learning theory that highlight the congruence between the two perspectives. This is followed by a description of the FROGI model and its application to a case scenario. I end with strategies for developing holistic presence.

What is Gestalt?

I have been writing about Gestalt for many years and when I think back, it seems everything about Gestalt if not outright radical, is unorthodox. Of course, context is important to understanding Gestalt's nonconformist ways. Gestalt began at the turn of the 19th century when revolutionary ideas took shape in all realms of society. One significant idea stemmed from a *theory of learning* put forth by German philosopher Graf Christian von Ehrenfels in the early 1900s. Von Ehrenfels coined the term "Gestalt," a German word loosely translated as form, configuration or whole. He believed his students learned best when they organized and considered concepts in their entirety rather than broken into individual parts. His learning theory caught the attention of three researchers at Berlin University – Kurt Wertheimer, Wolfgang Kohler and Kurt Koffka – who wanted to explore whether the brain has similar self-organizing tendencies that influence human perception. The question was if the brain sees only part of an object, does it naturally seek to see the complete object. Their research findings convinced them that the answer was yes. What followed for the three researchers was the founding of an unconventional perspective known as Gestalt psychology. Kurt Lewin, Fritz Perls and Laura Perls were members of the network of what I label the "radical Gestalt" at Berlin University at the time.

A few thoughts emerge about my sense of the "radical Gestalt."

Gestalt...
- defied isolationist theory and asserted holism;
- dared to challenge Freudian psychology and assumptions of Newtonian physics;
- applied mindfulness in the concept of "awareness" to the therapeutic process;
- created a relational and dialogic practice built on *use-of-self, presence* and *high contact;*
- focused on *now* when the world wanted to hold tight to *then* and *next;*
- prioritized *how* and *what* over *why;*
- considered the body a valid source of information in therapeutic practice;
- encouraged client responsibility and accountability;
- proclaimed *"resistance is good"* and *"change is paradoxical;"*
- formulated a systems theory of human behavior;
- positioned the group as a foundational and potent structure for social change;
- recognized the validity of learning from subjective experience.

The point I seek to underscore is from the initial backdrop of learning theory two paths central to Gestalt practice were shaped: one by Lewin who almost single handedly created the field of social psychology and in like manner influenced the founding of the field of organization development (OD); the other by Fritz Perls, Laura Perls, Isadore From and Paul Goodman who founded Gestalt therapy. Experiential Leaning Theory (Kolb, 1984) shares ancestral roots with Gestalt with an uncharacteristic perspective of holism and democracy in learning that aims to nullify the assumption of one best way to learn.

Intervening from a Gestalt Perspective: "Managing the Splash"

> The word Gestalt is a noun and a verb, suggesting both an end state and a process; thus, the Gestalt practitioner is constantly 'gestalting' in search of a fuller 'gestalt.'

Gestalt is a unique paradigm. Practitioners often hear from clients that they cannot describe what they do, adding they only know they experience something different. We explain that in the midst of complexity, our job is to "manage the splash." I often muse that the Gestalt practitioner is like a duck "paddling beneath the water." To the client, we appear to move smoothly across the turbulent streams of change that are full of stops and starts, sharp turns, and steep waves; but we are very busy and more often than not, uncertain about impact. The perceived composure is achieved by staying grounded and using foundational principles and methods of Gestalt that help keep the "splash" under control (see Rainey Tolbert, 2004 for details of Gestalt Organisation & Systems Development).

A. **Pursue Holism.** Rooted in self-organizing and social constructionist tendencies in human perception, the goal of Gestalt is to seek as full a picture as possible of the client situation. Lewin's field theory (Wulf, 1996, p. 3) is a behavioral parallel of general systems theory where he describes the interdependence between the organism (person, client) and the environment (environment or total field). Even when there is a client of one, the interest is as much about all that surrounds that one client and the nature of the interaction of the client with different parts of their context.

B. **Focus on Process.** Unlike typical intervention approaches where emphasis is on content and *what* work gets done, Gestalt tilts toward process and *how* work gets done. The task always at hand is noticing patterns and emerging themes: what is present and what is not present; connections and disconnections; what works well and what is challenging; who is with whom and who is not with anyone.

C. **Work from Awareness.** Chidiac (2018) portrays Gestalt practitioners as "awareness agents" rather than "change agents" while Siminovitch urges development of "awareness IQ" (2017). Their sentiments are aligned with the emphasis Gestalt places on consciously knowing in the moment – one way to describe awareness. It is a form of mindful attentiveness that supports the practitioner taking residence in what philosopher Salomon Friedlander describes as the "zone of indifference" or zero point where complexity, chaos and conflict can best be held (Wulf, 1996, p.3). This also allows relaxation of ego and need "to get it right."

D. **Bound Awareness.** Shape, organize, and configure awareness through the process of bounding to determine how and where to intervene. Boundaries – open or closed, broad or narrow, deep or shallow – influence the strength of connection or "contact" with self and others. A leader is aware that operations are too complex and change is needed. She bounds her awareness when she decides where best to launch the change – with the senior leadership team, the entire company, or the division that most or least exemplifies the desired vision.

E. **Transform Use-of-Self into Compelling Presence with High Contact.** Gestalt reframes use-of-self in the concept of "presence." Nevis (1987) states that not only does the practitioner "stand for and express certain values, attitudes, and skills, but to use these in a way to stimulate, and perhaps evoke from the client, action necessary for movement on its problems" (p.54). As such, presence becomes relational use-of-self through evocation or provocation. Engagement and high contact are essential. The practitioner is alert and internally and externally aware, energetically available and fluidly responsive to the client (Chidiac, 2018).

F. **Use the Cycle of Experience (CoE).** First outlined by Perls (1947), the CoE is a model for tracking real-time, here-and-now phenomena through a seven-phase cycle that can be applied to a range of experience – personal, coaching, conflict, group, or large-scale change.
   1. *Sensation.* Using the senses to gather data about self, others and the environment.
   2. *Awareness.* Noticing emergence of patterns and themes from the sensory data.
   3. *Energy.* Tracking energy and interest or lack thereof in the patterns and themes.
   4. *Action.* Transforming energy, interest, and excitement into action.
   5. *Contact.* Attending to the shifts and changes that occur as a result of action.
   6. *Closure.* Assessing achievements, highlighting learning, and celebrating success.
   7. *Withdrawal.* Supporting the need for rest, being, and renewal.

G. **Follow the Unit of Work (UoW).** While the CoE tracks here-and-now process, UoW is used to map, design, and organize planned change in three simple phases that overlay the CoE:
   1. *Beginning* (sensation, awareness). Determine the work.

2. *Middle* (mobilization of energy, action, contact.) Do the work.
3. *End* (closure, withdrawal). Close the work.

With a UoW, large interventions (macro goals) can proceed in smaller, manageable steps (micro tasks).

H. **Attend to Resistance.** It is rare that a client moves uninhibited through the CoE and UoW.

Often, the reason for working with a behavioral professional is to get "unstuck." The Gestalt practitioner comes prepared to work with "stuck systems," whether in the form of the pull and push of resistance, ambivalence, conflict, polarities, multiple realities or understanding the difference between a *problem to be solved* and *a dilemma to be managed*.

I. **Design Gestalt Experiments.** These are "on demand" learning experiences used to stimulate client awareness. Experiments are co-created by client and practitioner and enacted in the moment. The power of the Gestalt experiment lies in what is known as creating a "safe emergency." For instance, in the presence of the practitioner, two parties in conflict agree to "try new behavior" that involves some level of risk, yet is safe enough because of the trust they have in the practitioner.

Experiential Learning Theory

"What is essential is not that the therapist learn something about the patient and then teach it to him, but that the therapist teach the patient how to learn about himself (Perls, Hefferline and Goodman (1951, pp. 15-16)."

My introduction to experiential learning came during my graduate studies when I participated in my first T (training) – group. However, knowledge of the theoretical underpinnings of experiential earning did not arrive until my post graduate days at Case Western Reserve University "Case" in Cleveland, Ohio. During my first year, I was a teaching assistant to David Kolb in a course designed around experiential learning. It was also about this time that I became immersed in Gestalt theory and practice at the Gestalt Institute of Cleveland. Soon, the congruence between experiential learning and Gestalt became apparent. Holism and learning from experience were common and made for a natural fit for me personally.

In ELT, learning is portrayed as an idealized learning cycle or spiral where immediate *concrete experience* of sensations and feelings is the basis for *reflective observation* of themes and patterns that are assimilated through *abstract conceptualization* that are guides for *active experimentation*, application and practice. In ELT, there is no preferred way to learn, no learning hierarchy. Learning thus becomes a more holistic, integrative, and democratic process where the learner "touches all four learning bases," alternating between grasping experience and transforming experience. (Figure A shows the experiential learning cycle).

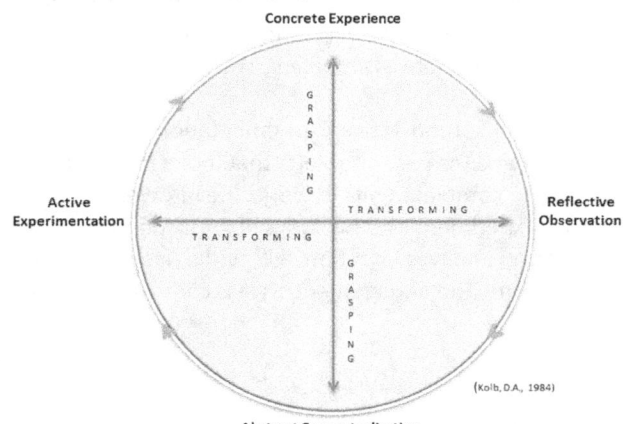

Figure A: The Experiential Learning Cycle

The FROGI Model

Claire Stratford introduced me to the original version of FROGI in the Gestalt International Organization & Systems Development Program (IOSD). She said she had received the idea from a student at Case. Claire would sketch the FROGI design on a sheet of paper. She did not make a fuss of too much. Soon, we began teaching the theory behind the model, refining it along the way. This is the first article that is devoted to the theory and practice of FROGI.

The Four Roles of the Gestalt Intervener framework is a simple and straight forward guide for practitioners working with complex dynamics. It translates the four modes of learning in ELT into four corresponding ways to intervene, providing more intervention options; thereby expanding the practitioner's range of presence.

- In *experiencing,* using Concrete Experience (CE), the focus is *the practitioner's* personal and immediate concrete experience. This involves an internal scan of sensory functions – see, hear, touch, smell and taste and the clearest guide for use-of-self. The engagement style is *role model.*
- In *noticing,* using Reflective Observation (RO), the practitioner observes patterns and themes emerging *from client behavior and immediate environment.* The focus is the client's process and dynamics. The engagement style is *process facilitator.*
- In *grand theorizing,* using Abstract Conceptualization (AC), the practitioner uses abstract theories, concepts, generalizations and metaphors to make-meaning of what is noticed *from the client and immediate environment.* The engagement style is *interpreter.*
- In *influencing,* using Active Experimentation (AE), the practitioner aims to create shifts that move the client around the CoE to complete units of work. The intervention could be a Gestalt experiment or other ways of impacting the work. Influencing involves intention, will, and a desire to help, guide and support. The engagement style is *coach and advisor.*

Case Scenario

The Executive Committee (ExCom) of a major multi-national firm meets to prepare a 30-minute presentation for the Board of Trustees. The focus of the presentation are the findings of the recent stakeholder satisfaction survey. The stakes are high because year-over-year performance numbers continue a downward trend in most areas of the company.

After contracting with the group about her role and the group's specific goals, the Gestalt practitioner positions herself at the table with the group so that she can effectively observe behavior and process; yet, not be a distraction. Grounding herself in awareness, she stays mindful of her internal experience while tracking behavioral dynamics (using the Cycle of Experience), task dynamics (using Unit of Work) as well as attending to the broader environmental context of the meeting (room, temperature, lighting, etc.). She then is prepared to use the FROGI model.

These are her observations after 20 minutes:
- Only half the group has participated in the discussion.

- The conflict between the Vice President (VP) of sales and the VP of manufacturing is being played out as the practitioner recalls it does each time the group meets.
- Her energy has begun to wane.
- Members of the group keep going in and out of the meeting to take calls.
- She has some idea of what might be happening in the group.
- She has thoughts about how to support the group's process.
- The group never seems to be able to make a decision that everyone supports.
- She notices a difference in the conversation when the more silent individuals participate.

Table 1 describes the practitioner's intervention choices.

Table 1: Case Scenario: Choosing a FROGI Intervention

Learning Mode	Intervener Role	Interventions
Concrete Experience	Experiencing	Practitioner discloses here-and-now personal experience. Example. "I am aware of how low my energy is as I listen to your conversation."
Reflective Observation	Noticing	Practitioner shares observations of patterns of behavior and themes emerging in the group. Example: "I notice that most of the time, everyone is not included in your conversation."
Abstract Conceptualization	Grand Theorizing	Offers a grand theory to help the group make meaning of their experience. Example: "When you include everyone, your decision-making process improves."
Active Experimentation	Influencing	Using the CoE and UoW, intervenes to advance the work. Examples: • Make a suggestion: "Be more inclusive in your decision-making." • Encourage dialogue and connection: "Talk among yourselves about your decision-making process." • Design a Gestalt Experiment: "Would you like to experience what it is like when everyone participates in decision-making?" • To the two VPs in conflict, "talk to each other about when you have been really effective in presenting to the Board of Trustees."

1. She determines the FROGI intervention that might be most helpful based on her "read" of the situation: experiencing, noticing, grand theorizing, or influencing.
2. She selects a level of system of the intervention: individual, two-person, sub-group, or total system.
3. She remembers the Gestalt intervention principle: *Clear. Concise. Get in. Get out.*

4. She makes her intervention, stays in awareness as she notices the impact, and begins the process all over again.
5. The goal is not to assess whether an intervention is right or wrong; rather, it is to assess if the intervention was carried out with clarity of intent. That is, did the practitioner do what she planned to do?

Feedback on FROGI

Generally, the FROGI gets good reviews when introduced to clients or in Gestalt education and training programs. Descriptions include "simple," "pragmatic," "accessible" and "fun." One corporate CEO described the framework as "delicious." However, there are points of feedback in each role worth mentioning.

- Experiencing can prove difficult for practitioners who customarily are detached and disconnected from themselves and others. The role directs awareness to the inner self, others and the immediate environment and requires the practioner to selectively disclose that awareness as an intervention. This is not an easy role to acquire for abstract learners.
- In Noticing, the art of pattern recognition is critical for it is where experience is organized into themes and "Gestalts." Practitioners must manage the tendency to interpret or judge rather than stay with data. Action-prone practitioners must acquire a taste for slowing down.
- Grand Theorizing is the most popular role. Initially, Gestalt faculty assumed the reason is it involves analytical skills. What was learned is that practitioners appreciate that after years of "bashing," abstract learning is again valued and has a place in process consultation. Clients say Grand Theorizing helps them "understand the madness" in their world.
- Some practitioners are confused by Influencing, believing that they should not "tell" the client what to do. Though initially challenged, practitioners are open to learning how to positively influence process, design Gestalt experiments, and make good contact.

Dual Learning Cycles in Relationship

We are often asked why the process begins with the intervener in the first role, then shifts to the client and environment in the other three roles. The individual learner is the focus of ELT. This is in contrast with the FROGI model which is a relational frame that attends to the interaction between intervener and client. Both client and intervener are moving around respective learning cycles except the intervener's cycle of learning is more background while the client's cycle of learning is foreground. The FROGI model very explicitly and intentionally begins with the practitioner's self as instrument but immediately shifts to the client. It is useful to remember only the individual can report their personal experience. Others can only notice and perceive another person's behavior.

Holistic Presence

Holistic presence is the combination of intervening from a Gestalt perspective using basic principles and methods of Gestalt, e.g., Cycle of Experience, Unit of Work and the Four Roles of the Intervener (Figure B). Practitioners should become knowledgeable of experiential learning theory. This involves learning how to learn, becoming familiar with the experiential learning cycle, their personal learning preferences, and learning flexibility. All are useful in guarding against bias and overuse of a particular role (Kolb & Kolb, 2005a). This can be achieved by administering the Kolb Learning Style Inventory (Kolb & Kolb, 2011).

Figure B:
Elements of Holistic Presence: CoE, UoW, and FROGI

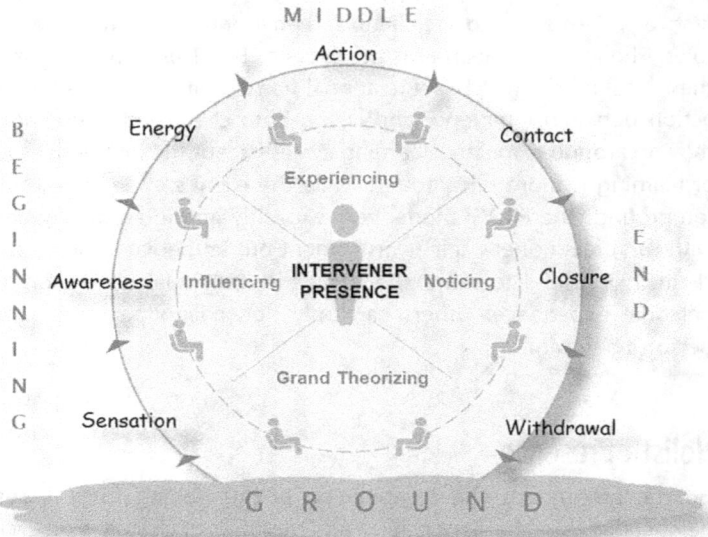

Cultivating Holistic Presence

Immediate steps for cultivating holistic presence are outlined below and includes suggestions from Yeganeh and Kolb (2009) on mindful practice in each role.

Developing capacity for Experiencing (CE). Clearing the mind is central to engaging in present moment experience. Deep breathing anchors the mind in immediate, here-and-now sensorial awareness of sight, sound, touch, taste, and smell. Suggested practices include meditation and mindfulness that also reduce stress, increase clarity and calmness, and improve health. Interpersonal skills such as leadership, relationship and giving and receiving feedback can improve by developing the experiencing role.

Developing capacity for Noticing (RO). Observing behavioral dynamics and processes without judgement or interpretation is essential. Noticing can be enhanced by deliberately viewing things from different perspectives and with empathy. Stillness and quieting the mind fosters the ability to notice. This allows patterns and themes

"Gestalts" to surface. Noticing expands ability to appreciate multiple realities and engenders a natural tendency for diversity and inclusion. Information skills of pattern and theme recognition, data management and analysis can aid in noticing.

Developing capacity for Grand Theorizing (AC). Questioning assumptions can help focus the mind to make "theories-in-use" intentional rather than automatic. Taking time to view the relationship among themes and behavioral patterns can enrich grand theories. Creating contextual and relational knowledge rather than pursuing dichotomous thinking strengthens the capacity for grand theorizing. Analytical skills of theory building, data analysis and technology management can aid in the development and expression of grand theories.

Developing capacity for Influencing (AE). In influencing, the practitioner moves into the practical world of real consequences for the client. Influencing can be enhanced by working on the ability to intervene gracefully, without distracting from the client's work. Practitioners can become competent in conducting Gestalt experiments by starting with less complicated experiments, such as Exaggeration (of behavior), Fantasy (imagining), and Language (e.g., use of "I" instead of "they") that allow practitioners to try, test, and evaluate generative actions that are not too complicated. Practitioners must resist the automatic self-judgments, self-schemas, feelings and thoughts that support tendencies not to influence. Often there is an assumption that influencing is bad. This can be overcome by accepting influencing as a critical part of Gestalt work. Action skills, initiative, goal setting, and action taking, help in developing performance mastery.

Summary

As the world searches for novel ideas and innovative technologies to cope with change and complexity, the need for adaptive processes at the basic human level must not be forgotten. Learning is essential. With the FROGI model, Gestalt finds a partner in learning that elevates Gestalt practice to a fresh platform of contemporary knowledge and practice. Based on Kolb's experiential leaning theory, FROGI enhances the practitioner's ability to development holistic presence in four ways: (1) be fully in the moment through experiencing (2) attend to the client's experience and broader environment through noticing, (3) make meaning of and clarify that experience by grand theorizing, and (4) through influencing, support the client actively, creatively, and expediently testing and trying innovative ways of not only responding to but anticipating environmental demands.

References

Beisser, A. (1970). The Paradoxical Theory of Change. In J. Fagan and L. Shepherd, ed., *Gestalt Therapy Now*. Palo Alto: Science and Behavior Books.

Chidiac, MA. (2018). *Relational Organisational Gestalt: An Emergent Approach to Organisation Development*. New York: Routledge.

Kolb, A. Y. & Kolb, D. A. (2017). The Experiential Educator: Principles and Practices of Experiential Learning. Kaunakakai, HI: EBLS Press.

Kolb, D. A. (2015) Experiential learning: Experience as the source of learning and development. 2nd Edition. Upper Saddle River NJ: Pearson Education.

Kolb, A. Y. & Kolb, D. A. (2011). Learning Style Inventory Version 4.0 Korn Ferry/Hay Group Retrieved from: http://store.kornferry.com/store/lominger/en_US/list/categoryID.4836644000/parentCategoryID.4836643700.

Buckingham, M. & Goodall, A. (2019). The feedback fallacy. Harvard Business Review. March-April, pp. 92-101. Retrieved from: https://hbr.org/2019/03/the-feedback-fallacy.

Nevis, E. (1987). *Organizational Consulting: A Gestalt Approach*. New York: Gardner Press.

Perls, F.S. (1947) Ego, Hunger and Aggression. Gouldsboro, MD: Gestalt Journal Press.

Perls, F.S., Hefferline, R. & Goodman, P. (1951) Gestalt therapy. New York: Julian Press.

Rainey, MA; Jones, B. (2014). Use of Self as an OD Practitioner. In: B. Jones and M. Brazzel, Eds. *The NTL Handbook of Organisation Development and Change, Second Edition*. San Francisco: Pfeiffer.

Rainey, M. A., Hekelman, F., Galazka, S.F., & Kolb, D. A. (1993, February). Job demands and personal skills in family medicine: Implications for faculty development. Family Medicine, 25, 100–103.

Rainey, M. A., & Kolb, D. A. (1995). Using experiential learning theory and learning styles in diversity education. In R. R. Sims & S. J. Sims (Eds.), The importance of learning styles: Understanding the implications for learning, course design and education (pp. 129–46). Westport, CT: Greenwood Press.

Rainey, M.A. & Kolb, D.A. (2014). Leading in a learning way. In B. B. Jones & M. Brazzel (Eds.), (2014). *The NTL Handbook of Organization Development and Change: Principles, Practices, Perspectives* (2nded.). San Francisco: Wiley.

Rainey Tolbert, M.A. (2004). What is Gestalt organization & systems development? All about the O, the S, the D…and of course, Gestalt. *OD Practitioner*, Vol. 36, No.4, (pp. 6-10).

Siminovitch, D. E. (2017). A Gestalt Primer: The Path toward Awareness IQ. Gestalt Coaching Works, LLC: USA.

Wilson, A. L. & Hayes, E. R. (2002). From the Editors: The problem of (learning in-from-to experience) experience. Adult Education Quarterly. 52(3): 173-175.

Wulf, R. (1996) The historical roots of Gestalt therapy theory. (pp. 1-9)

Retrieved from http://www.gestalt.org/wulf.htm. Originally appeared in the November, 1996, issue of *Gestalt Dialogue: Newsletter for the Integrative Gestalt Centre*, New Zealand.

Yeganeh, B. & Kolb, D. (2009). Mindfulness and experiential learning. In OD Practitioner, 41, 3, 8-14.

III. GESTALT PRACTICE AT MULTIPLE LEVELS OF SYSTEM

Chapter 6: Navigating the Inner Emotional Landscape in a Globalized World

Eva Roettgers

Are we living in really special times or is it only our perception that something unusual is going on in our own life and work worlds – even in the world at large? I frequently hear friends and colleagues bemoan, "I feel unsettled. I am in a transition. I do not know what will come next." I often read the same sentiment in blogs and newspapers. For many, daily life is routine: They are raising kids, working, meeting friends and enjoying family. However, for many others there is uneasiness or even fear about what is going on in their worlds. If their lives are undergoing a big transition, they are excited about promising new opportunities or feel threatened by an uncertain future.

We are undeniably experiencing large-scale changes – technologically, environmentally, economically, culturally and politically. But are these changes more intense and of greater magnitude than we have experienced during the past 70 years or are we merely more aware of the increasing complexity in the larger environment? And does that have a direct effect on our state of mind and behaviors, regardless of our country, religion, gender, class, age or profession?

Gestalt psychology answers these questions by viewing the way we process information as a holistic phenomenon: perception of the whole is radically different from the perception of its component parts.

> "Gestalt psychology is an attempt to understand the laws behind the ability to acquire and maintain meaningful perceptions in an apparently chaotic world. The central principle of Gestalt psychology is that the mind forms a <u>global whole</u> with self-organizing tendencies." [*]

> "Gestalt psychologists have sought to understand the organization of cognitive processes.... Our brain is capable of generating whole forms, particularly with respect to the visual

---

[*] "Gestalt Psychology," n.d., para. 1)

> *recognition of global figures instead of just collections of simpler and unrelated elements (points, lines, curves, etc.)."* *

In the Gestalt approach, we see the human organism as a self-regulating entity with the need to open and close its boundaries towards the environment for an exchange in order to stay alive. At the contact boundary of the organism-environment field, polarized forces are seen as drivers for this exchange and regulators of opening up and closing down process.

Gestalt as a holistic approach opens our horizon for a systemic perspective: the Gestalt model does not solely consider an individual as a dynamic integrated organism, but also other human systems such as groups, teams, organizations, nations, etc. Applying Gestalt principles to larger "wholes" help us to see how "themes and conflicting needs" or "polarized forces" on one level of a human system are expressed on other levels of the system. This is a sort of holographic phenomena.

Polarities in organizations can be addressed by:
- Integrating the polarities to create a synergetic system;
- Ignoring or even deleting one polarity with presumptive negative effects;
- Organizing the polarities in a hierarchical order, e.g.: "one is more important than the other."

A healthy organization needs a "living equilibrium" of contradicting needs before it can achieve pre-defined goals and allow space and time for learning. These tensions can be perceived at different levels of system. For example, for the individual, tension could appear when making decisions such as how to use available time for learning, making money or both. For the organization, questions about investing in education as a collective and learning for the good of everybody could drive the tension, especially if challenged to consider factors such as, does "common sense" dictate that learning is mainly an individual decision and needs to be done outside of work time with own resources?

For centuries, cultures, nations, organizations, individuals have developed mechanisms to deal with inherent polarities of human life and to find creative solutions to adapt to a changing environment. Is there a significant difference nowadays? The perception is that the tensions between the polarities and their awareness on a large scale are increasing exponentially on all levels: globally, within nations, in companies, in individuals. The need for understanding the information processing mechanisms and the effects

---

* "Gestalt Psychology," n.d.

of increasing tensions on human systems is growing as they can generate energies for transformative developments for humanity or create fragmentation and destructive tendencies with potential negative outcomes.

This chapter wants to build on the Gestalt body of knowledge about perception and information processing and offers a map for understanding our capacity to digest the increasing complexity of the internal and external environment. The map will enable us to navigate through our inner physical, emotional and mental landscape on an individual and collective level in a VUCA-world (volatility, uncertainty, complexity, ambiguity). From my coaching and consulting experiences, this map has enabled people to broaden their perception of reality and to allow new choices. This is especially relevant for organizations where digitalization, acceleration of changes and disruptive developments require new approaches. This model supports ways of dealing constructively with stuck states and all kinds of human defense mechanisms.

Information Processing Systems from the Perspective of Gestalt Concepts and Recent Brain Research

The Gestalt Approach focuses on the boundary where exchange takes place. Every organism lives by digesting, assimilating and integrating something new whether it is food, experiences, information, influences, conflicts, ideas or theories. Thus, the organism is able to reproduce, preserve and grow itself. This process requires adapting "new" elements by perceiving what is digestible and what is not and decomposing existing forms into assimilable or integrable elements.

One of the main membranes to the outer world is the human brain. Our senses and nerves supply our brain with about 20 million bits of information from the internal and external stimuli every second. The brain processes information as physical, emotional and mental signals and impulses for acting, relating, talking and responding. As we are exposed to a multitude of data at the same time, for example an internal signal for "hunger", noises from a construction site and, and, and…., the brain had to develop a mechanism to avoid being paralyzed by a data overload. Thus, only a few elements of the incoming data become conscious, while the rest will be digested subconsciously*. And by growing up, we learn how to organize this information processing.

---

* Some researchers say 95% of internal and external data are processed unconsciously.

Neurological Development of Human Information Processing System

Among mammals, humans have a long socialization process, which means they are not able to survive socialization period without social caring. Openness for incoming data and learning how to deal with all the information is crucial for early childhood development. Observing very small children, we can see that they will take in data without filters and their reactions will be direct and instantaneous. Although some instinctual reactions and extraordinary robustness are "built in", little children have limited capacities to differentiate what is okay and what is not okay. They can become easily overwhelmed by too much data or being exposed to critical situations. Hopefully, their caretakers will ensure that they are protected from serious threats to their lives.

Growing up is mainly a learning process to gain autonomy, self-empowerment, adaptability to changing circumstances, capabilities for self-protection and connecting to the social environment. As we grow older, we develop a semi-permeable boundary as a result of our experiences and received teachings. We learn to open up when it is appropriate and to close down by reducing our contact to the environment as a protection mechanism. This is mainly an unconscious, physical process of relaxation and contraction accompanied by emotional and mental equivalents.

As grownups, our brain has developed specific processing mechanisms for incoming information. First, it will scan incoming data and its interpretation follows a clear hierarchy of needs. Protection of one's physical existence has absolute priority. Initially, an instinctive and quick decision is made unconsciously, based on stored past experiences of safety or danger. If...
- a signal for danger is identified, an emergency program of heightened alertness or reaction will kick-in within milliseconds
- nothing is flagged, the data will be processed slower and more differentiated.

Depending on incoming signals, our "psychic immune system" regulates whether we open up or close down to whatever happens around us and within our body. This system works automatically to ensure that our life will be secure and vibrant with relatively easy adaptive responses to whatever circumstances we are in.

At the **organism-environment boundary,** information will be channeled through the "data scanner" of our organism. Depending on the decoding of the signals, different degrees of permeability are triggered:
- If this self-regulation mechanism of opening-up and closing-down is flexible and dynamic, the system has access to information and resources of the outer and inner environment, resulting in a "living equilibrium" of a healthy system
- If all types of non-filtered data are entering, the system is in constant overload with a high probability of collapsing
- If it is more or less closed to external impulses, the system has to draw upon its own inner resources, and in a long run it simply dies.

Different Zones of our "psychic immune system"

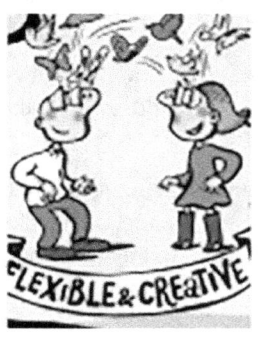

Zone of open mindedness with an "agile mindset" for learning and growth. In a state of openness, we can consciously hold all kinds of perspectives, polarities and data without identifying and needing to act upon them. When I am relaxed, my attitude towards whatever happens in and around me is characterized by interest and curiosity. Depending on the 'newness' of the stimuli this could be accompanied with excitement and insecurity without interrupting the "approach posture". The field of open-mindedness is the space of potentiality, creativity, possibilities, resources, unknown territory. It is the field of experiments, new challenges, new options and choices. In this stage a variety of emotions, body sensations, mental activities are conscious and. If mindfulness and reflective behavior are in the foreground, we are able to face a huge amount of data and the increasing complexity in our environment without feeling overwhelmed. On the other hand, this wide open awareness might lead to an experience of "opening a Pandora's Box" – past experiences that are buried in the unconsciousness are showing up with the challenge to hold it without repeating the same behavior and emotions of the original experience.

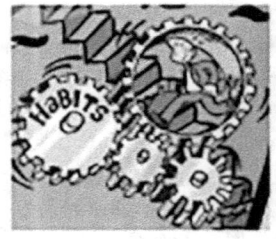
Comfort Zone of habits and beliefs, based on past experiences, to stay safe in familiar circumstances. When we rely on proven habits and beliefs, our body "rewards" us with feelings of well-being by disposing of "dopamine and endogenous opiates." Stored behavioral routines and beliefs can be retrieved easily and fast by autopilot. When I get into the car, I don't have to think about how driving works, it's stored in my whole body. I can drive a car and have a lively conversation at the same time. In order not to disturb these routines, the mind has well-suitable tools like mottos "Don't touch a running system" or "Only facts, no feelings". By blocking all data that contradict my habits and conviction and by being with people of a similar mindset and doing activities I feel competent in, I increase the comfort in my daily life. Polarities are being "handled" by differentiating what is "good and bad", "right and wrong", "first and then" with a clear either-or-decision.

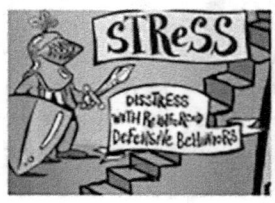
Stress Zone where our body provides additional energy to address actual challenges.

If something happens in the environment, which is perceived as strange or hostile, stress reactions are activated by providing additional energy. For example, an office worker looks forward to meeting a friend at 7:00 pm. Just as he is about to leave the office, he receives a call from his boss asking for a presentation to be done by tomorrow morning. Suddenly we have a mind-body-reaction, the adrenaline goes up, emotions like anger raise. "No, I'm not going to do that, I have a right to leave work!" Or, "Maybe I can do it, if I work fast and do a quick and dirty version", or doubts arise, such as "What could happen, if I do not do it?" These polarized, internal needs cause physical, emotional and mental stress with the perception an immediate response would be required. Stress reactions are helpful in mobilizing instant energy, but do not support taking time for decision making. They can become a problem if the person is not aware of the pressure, the inner conflicts are not explicitly addressed, or the person feels paralyzed between the different needs. If these experiences are repeated again and again, it can lead to somatic symptoms and eventually to a burnout.

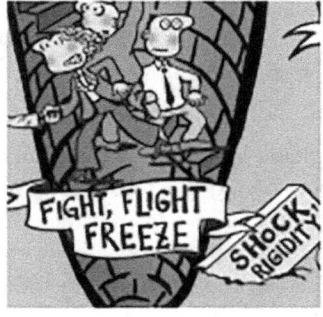

Survival Zone where all energies are mobilized within an instant when our instincts signal our life is in danger. If a person or a system gets into a life-threatening situation, instinctual fight-flight-freeze responses will be triggered, mobilizing all energies to generate necessary defense reactions. As this is a very adequate body response, for some people this experience of feeling overwhelmed by a sudden, out-of-control event can become a serious problem. This happens if the realization that the event is over does not take place and incoming data are chronically perceived as similarly life threatening. It is a reaction like a "record with a crack" repeating only a certain part of the song over and over again with the only choice between the extreme polarities of "live or die". The person is caught in a vicious circle of trauma responses which can lead to addiction or serious illness.

Creative Adaption as a Human Capacity – Openness, Comfort, Stress and Survival Zones

Having described these neurobiological mechanisms, how can they help us understand and adapt to our increasingly complex environment? The states we have described – openness, comfort, stress and survival zone – are helpful, necessary and make sense when dealing with the challenges of daily life. The question is: How can we as individuals remain fluid between the different zones in face of the increasing complexity of our world? Or as the goal of Gestalt therapy describes it *".... to become more fully and creatively alive and to become free from the blocks and unfinished business that may diminish satisfaction, fulfillment, and growth, and to experiment with new ways of being"*[*] The idea is not to stay all the time in the zone of openness, learning and development.

There are situations where automatic behaviour patterns make a lot of sense, such as:
- driving a car without having to think where the brakes are, how do I steer in the left direction, etc.

---

* "Gestalt Psychology," n.d.)

- walking in the woods where wild boars live and cautious behaviour is appropriate.
- being able to run to catch the bus, so that you arrive on time for a concert

Unfortunately, people could lose this fluidity. Automatic reactivity fuelled out of unconscious patterns is dominating our responses. We could become more or less stuck, for example, in the "comfort zone". The need for feeling secure might dominate many of our activities. Beliefs, habits and behaviours, experienced in the past that ensured safety, will be consciously or unconsciously our favourite choices. We justify them as the "right" and "the only way" without allowing a moment of consideration of other options. Or impulses of our internal or external environment trigger constant feelings of stress or even posttraumatic stress responses – an endless repetition of a threatening situations, experienced in the past. A healthy individual is present in his/her life with an attitude of openness for what is happening and is able to shift to behaviours of another layer, according to the changes in the internal or external environment.

Strategies that support this fluidity:
- **Relaxation, relaxation, relaxation**: When I am in a relaxed state, I open up physically, emotionally and mentally. This allows me to become aware of new stimuli in a calm, neutral way. Even when my learned reaction of attraction or repulsion shows up, I can be aware of it without an instant judgment of good or bad or a habit of "what is wrong attention" with the corresponding routines and stress reactions. The antidote to automatic defence reactivity would be to slow down, to sense what is happening in our body, feel the ground under our feet, breathe and stay in touch with what is present. The more we develop different ways to soothe ourselves and get back to a relaxed physiological state, the easier it is to experience the state of open-mindedness and fluid movements between the different zones.
- **Awareness, awareness, and awareness:** To see, hear, sense, smell, taste as much as possible with a wide-angle lens observing what is happening in my internal and external environment. This intensified contact with reality in the here-and-now leads to an experience of a constant information flow. Reflecting about the incoming data can help us know our trigger for high arousal reactions or "amygdala hijacks" without needing to react. This leads to more chances of discovering

choices and support within the environment. When the awareness of the here-and-now is reduced, proven, familiar solutions from the past seem to be appropriate for today. Our thoughts move to past or future events and narrow the available potential of what the environment has to offer in this moment.
- **Change to an "Approach State" and train your ability to shift between different zones:** By increasing our awareness, we can identify if we act out of our comfort zone or with a stress reaction or even feel trapped in a victim-perpetrator-reaction formation. By reflecting on the context, we might see what triggered our closing down reaction is based in memories of the past. Addressing the "old Gestalt" and separating the "here-and-now" conditions from the "then-and-there" situation might help to widen our horizon and increase our ability to choose between a variety of scenarios.

Once, we feel relaxed, open for the unknown and remain flexible, also in new, unfamiliar and even extreme situations, we can access the space of potentialities and possibilities.

The Holistic Approach: Application for Larger Systems

In the business world, new technological and social developments require innovations as well as the ability to differentiate what we need to continue and what we need to change. Relying on familiar, proven products, processes and business models will not guarantee the future survival of an organization. Members of innovative startups get very excited about new opportunities and see big chances to grow into new, unknown fields. Even large corporations start risky experiments with disruptive business models. For companies, an open mindset of their executives and employees with the ability to be aware of the complex interconnectedness around us is seen as a requirement for their survival.

At the same time, there are predictions that up to 70% of actual jobs might be gone within the next years due to the artificial intelligence revolution. It is no surprise that anxiety and stress responses are rising on a large scale. Using the described map "Navigating the inner emotional landscape," we can differentiate organizational cultures dealing with these challenges along the different zones of the psychic immune system:
- **Startup cultures** have an agile mindset with widespread

GESTALT PRACTICE: LIVING AND WORKING IN PURSUIT OF WHOLISM

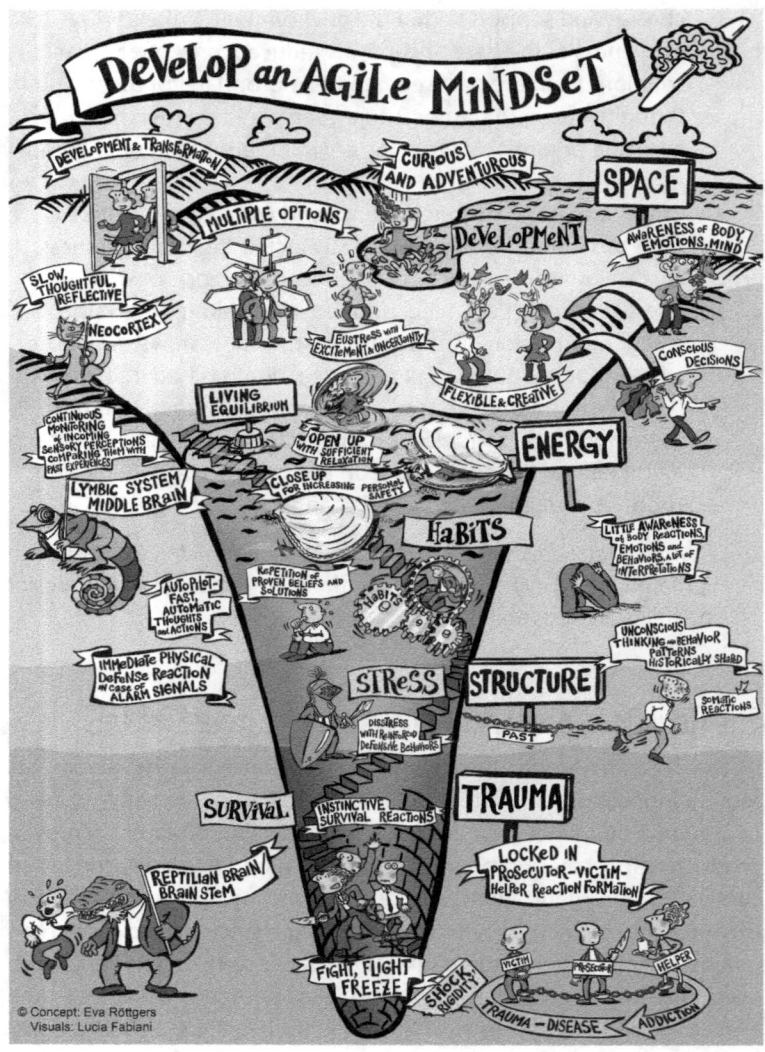

open-mindedness. This mindset can be described as enthusiastic, a risk-friendly attitude for entering new territories, high adaptability with fast pivots for new opportunities, intrinsic motivation as a drive for passionate engagement, a team approach with iterative, experiential learning cycles with continuous feedback, self-empowerment and working in networks with less hierarchical structures. Others would describe the effects as chaotic, more buzzwords than reality, reduced performance and cost consciousness, not predictable outcomes, more a playground than a serious business environment.

- **Bureaucratic organizations** are in contrast characterized by predictable procedures and routines to ensure the stability of the organization. Well-defined responsibilities in different functions are organized in silos, planning their next steps. Top-down-leadership style, limited engagement of employees and conflict avoidance are mechanisms to guarantee stable circumstances. If performance problems or a crisis cannot be ignored, individuals are made accountable for causing the trouble and/or being responsible for finding solutions.
- **Action-oriented organizational cultures** are in most cases very performance oriented with a high risk for stressful work conditions. Operative hectic with little prioritization along available resources, long-working hours often combined with a lot of work for the wastebasket, micromanagement leadership style, political games and power struggles between different interest groups, etc. are all a setup for burnout of their members. Escalation of conflicts to top management creates bottle-necks of decision taking. These organizations sometimes end up in a situation of a "rocking chair" – constant movement getting no-where.
- **Trapped organizations** are stuck in traumatic events in the organizational life cycle, like bankruptcy or a merger process. These organizations celebrate their "heroes" who are able to perform "last-minute-rescue-operations" without being aware that this need for fire-fighting might be due to internal dysfunctional patterns. Main issues are the missing cooperation of disintegrated parts of the company and an internal ignorance in face of important signals from the environment. If management asks for new solutions and taking risks, the "not possible" answer of direct reports are often justified by a story that happened long ago in the history of the company, e.g., where a manager was

fired because of making an error or failed with a new strategy. The whole company can be described as paralyzed, energies blocked, new ideas are encountered with a pessimistic outlook, people with talents and ambitions leave the company – a vicious circle with little light at the end of the tunnel.

Strategies of Healthy Organizations Dealing with Complexity in Our Environment

As we are in a transformational period we can see all kind of experiments and innovations of business models, organizational structures and culture. As countries, industries, professions, etc. are in different developmental phases with specific characteristics, each of these conditions different approaches might be suitable. There seems to be no one 'right' or 'wrong' model. Each organization has to find their own way for their development depending on the specific circumstances.

Different authors have described important qualities of a healthy organizational culture:

- **Dynamic Robustness** by oscillating between open-mindedness and reliable structures and processes with highly adaptive and resilient capabilities of their members. Contradicting polarities are seen as needed for the development of a system. They require constant balancing efforts, learning and communication about different needs of the involved stakeholders in order to find creative solutions which lead to thought-through decisions. High reliability organizations with Organizational Mindfulness are role models for the needed processes and structures (Weick & Sutcliffe, 2001).
- The **Gestalt Approach to Organizational Development** has been built on Kurt Lewin's change model "unfreeze-transform-refreeze", but the capability for not only one change effort, but a continuous creative adaption attitude is seen as one of the cornerstones of this approach. The Gestalt Cycle of Experience can be described as an iterative learning process with a diagnostic perspective to identify interruptions of the "contacting process", which block the fluidity of the process on different system levels. The knowledge and experiences about interventions on the intrapersonal, interpersonal and the level of the whole system provide a rich tool set for supporting healthy organizations in a fast-changing environment.

- **Leading from within with an open mind (curiosity), open heart (compassion) and open will (courage)** is the approach Otto Scharmer (2009) has developed with the Theory U where openness for new data and the wellbeing of the whole system is seen as a priority.
- *Corporate Life Cycles* (Adizes, 2004); *Developmental Stages in the Organizational Evolution* (Glasi and Lievegoed, 2004); *Becoming a Deliberately Developmental Organization* (Kegan and Lahey, 2016); *Spiral Dynamics* (Beck and Cowan, 2005); etc. – all these approaches see organizations in a developmental process with the potential of a growing capacity of the system to deal with the complexity of the environment.

Developments in Our Larger Context

In a world with an accelerated, increasing complexity, where the majority chooses unconsciously the path of closing down, the effects will be fragmentation, splitting and a slowed down development[*]:
- the gap between rich and poor seems to grow with different political approaches on how to address social inequality;
- the relationship between men and women, the MeToo movement and gender equality have become hot topics in the last years;
- the opinions about climate change vary – will it effects our region or far away regions like the South Pacific Islands or has the turning point already been crossed?
- the advances made through internet, social media, IT-technology, artificial intelligence are seen by some as a blessing for mankind, for others as means for a totalitarian surveillance state
- do we have a growing number of left-behind, marginalized parts of the population and a global elite which is busy in their limited bubble?
- do we care about migrants who had to leave their homes and countries because of war, poverty and climate change effects or do we think primarily of the welfare of our own people?

---

[*] Otto Scharmer (07 Nov. 2018) describes these phenomena in different countries in his article 'Axial Shift: The Decline of Trump, the Rise of the Greens, and the New Coordinates of Societal Changes.'

On a larger system level, all those phenomena are creating unprecedented tensions and pressures. Globalized interdependencies and its unpredictable consequences are shaking up political systems and socio-cultural relationships in many countries of the world. One view is that fragmentation and social divide will increase internal and external tensions and lead to escalating and irreconcilable confrontations within a society. Another movement we see, are all kind of activities to fight for the recognition of subgroups and liberation of individuals. Self-improving efforts, mindfulness training, coaching should provide support for individuals to thrive in a complex world but could turn paradoxically into mechanisms of defense reactions with limited effects.

For a holistic approach, integration of polarities and the well-being of the whole are the guiding principles. If members of a group, organization or community with different, even contradicting needs and opinions have an attitude of open mindedness and shared superordinate goals, there are chances to avoid fragmentation. By practicing dialogues, the involved people might be able to develop creative solutions instead of ignoring, shaming, hating, fighting or suppressing one pole. For these dialogues, we need to enhance our capacity to stay open in face of overwhelming complexity and contradicting opinions. We need to operate as empowered, autonomous individuals with agile mindsets in strong, dynamic collectives.

Promising approaches are the efforts of (local) communities, where members are committed to reflect and open themselves to enter unknown territories. Many organization – small or large, nonprofit or profit – are experimenting with the reduction and decentralization of hierarchical power structures and inviting their members to explore self-management and collective leadership. If we look at the model of the "psychic immune system", we understand the automatic response of many individuals in these unsettling times with the belief that a secure future will be possible through protection of borders, maintaining familiar circumstances and be part of a like-minded community. On the other hand, having confidence, trust and excitement about new opportunities would be – in my eyes – a more promising mindset. Accompanied with the capabilities:

- to stay in contact but grounded in an agitated world
- to trust that by embracing the inherent polarities and allow the dialogue between the different needs a next, meaningful step will show up
- to differentiate when it is safe to open up and when it makes sense to stick to proven processes and behaviors and when it is wise to protect one's vulnerability

- for resilience to go back to "normal" after an unsettling experience, we have what is needed to navigate our inner emotional landscape.

This is an individual and a collective learning and developmental process. If we as individuals and as collectives become conscious of our traditional neurological wiring with automatic defense responses this awareness might provide us with the capacity, willingness and competence to open ourselves up to the complex, paradoxical challenges we are all facing in a globalized world.

References

Adizes, I. (2004). *Managing Corporate Lifecycles – how organizations grow, age and die*. Santa Barbara, CA: The Adizes Institute Publishing.

Beck, D. E. & Cowan, C. C. (2005). *Spiral Dynamics: Mastering Values, Leadership and Change*. Oxford, UK: Blackwell Publishing.

'Gestalt Psychology.' (23 March 2018/19 March 2019). *Wikipedia: The Free Encyclopedia*. https://en.wikipedia.org/wiki/Gestalt_psychology.

Glasi, F. & Lievegoed, B. (2004). (3rd Ed.) *Dynamische Unternehmensentwicklung. Grundlegen fur nachhaltiges Change Management*. Bern/Stuttgart/Wien: Haupt Verlag.

Kegan, R. & Lahey, L. L. (2016). *An Everyone Culture: Becoming a Deliberately Developmental Organization*. Boston: Harvard Business Review Press.

Sharmer, C. O. (2009). *Theory U: Leading from the Future as it Emerges*. San Francisco: Berrett-Koehler.

Sharmer, C. O. 07 November 2018. 'Axial Shift: The Decline of Trump, the Rise of the Greens, and the New Coordinates of Societal Change'. *In the Field of the Future Blog*.

Retrieved from: *https://www.presencing.org/transforming-capitalism-lab/stories/axial-shift*.

Weick, K. E. & Sutcliffe, K. M. (2001). *Managing the Unexpected: Assuring High Performance in an Age of Complexity*. San Francisco: Jossey-Bass.

Chapter 7: Preventing the Tragedy of the Commons: A Call to Gestalt OD Practitioners to Pursue Holism for the Renewal of our Global Systems

Kate Cowie

Introduction

In the ancient stories of every culture, the Hero embarks on a journey into unknown places and, having reinvented himself in his battles with the fearsome creatures he encounters, he returns to his familiar land to bring about the collective renewal of his community (Campbell, 1993). When we encounter an enduring motif such as this we can be sure that it has served those who have gone before us in the primary activity of being human – meaning-making (Kegan, 1982, p.11). In recent decades, much has been written about the journey – the universal 'Search for Self', the search for who we are and, moreover, who we could be. Much less, however, has been written about the phenomenon of 'collective renewal'. What is the nature of it? And why and how should it be achieved?

This chapter is a contribution towards addressing this shortfall in an era of breakdown in our global systems. It asserts that individual and organisational development are conjoined (as the myths and legends of the past suggest), and that organisations, as essential elements of our new, interconnected world, are obligated to play their part in the necessary work of system transformation. It draws on the following theories as they are applied in the practice field of 'Gestalt' Organisation Development ('OD'):*

---

* The Gestalt approach to the discipline of Organisation Development (OD) blends the principles of Gestalt Psychology and Gestalt Therapy with the premises and practices of OD, enabling practitioners to take a holistic, integrated and optimistic stance as they collaborate with their clients to improve effectiveness at all levels of system (individual, interpersonal, group, organisation and society).

> *The Theory of Holism*: 'holism' is a term that was coined by JG Smuts in 1926 to designate the tendency in nature to produce wholes (bodies or organisms) from the ordered grouping of unit structures. The general principle of holism was articulated by the classical philosopher, Aristotle, in *The Metaphysics* thus: "The whole is more than the sum of the parts".
>
> *The Paradoxical Theory of Change:* Arnold Beisser, drawing on the work of Frederick Perls, proposed in 1970 that change occurs when one becomes what one is, not when one tries to becomes what one is not: "The premise is that one must stand in one place in order to have firm footing to move and that it is difficult or impossible to move without that footing".
>
> *General Systems Theory*: an interdisciplinary theory of organisation, founded by, amongst others, Ludwig von Bertalanffy in the late 1930s. His best-known contribution is his delineation of the characteristics of 'closed' and 'open' systems; in this frame of reference, an 'open' system is a complex of elements in mutual interaction, and in exchange with its environment.

And it calls on Gestalt OD practitioners to bring to bear their awareness, their skills and their insights to foster the development of Self, others and organisations, in order to prevent the 'tragedy of the commons'*, the destruction of our shared resource-systems by multiple users acting independently, according to their own self-interest, whilst neglecting the well-being of society as a whole.

---

* The concept of the 'Tragedy of the Commons' was articulated first by the British economist, William Forster Lloyd, in 1833 in his description of the effects of unregulated grazing on common land. 'Common land' is land over which a number of people, known as 'commoners', have 'rights of common' e.g. 'pasturage' (the right to graze livestock), 'pannage' (the right to put pigs out to feed in wooded areas) and 'turbary' (the right to take turf or peat for fuel). The concept was made popular by the American ecologist, Garrett Hardin, in an article in 1968. The over-exploitation of the 'commons' (any shared and unregulated resource) by individuals acting independently according to their own self-interest and without attention to the needs of all, is evident in many different contexts today. And, as the world's population rises and demands more access to the commons, our shared resource-systems are threatened with collapse.

CHAPTER 7: PREVENTING THE TRAGEDY OF THE COMMONS

The Human Adventure: the Pursuit of Holism

Our understanding of the human development journey is fundamental to our inquiry into the phenomenon of 'collective renewal'. It was first charted in earnest by the early sages and mystics who came forward from 1600 BCE. They described it as one of five stages of increasing *wholeness* ascending from matter, to life, to mind, to soul and ultimately to spirit. It is often illustrated as a nest of concentric spheres: each dimension incorporates components of its predecessor, and constitutes a new, higher – or more complex, more integrated, more differentiated – organisation (Wilbur, 2001).

The Great Nest of Being

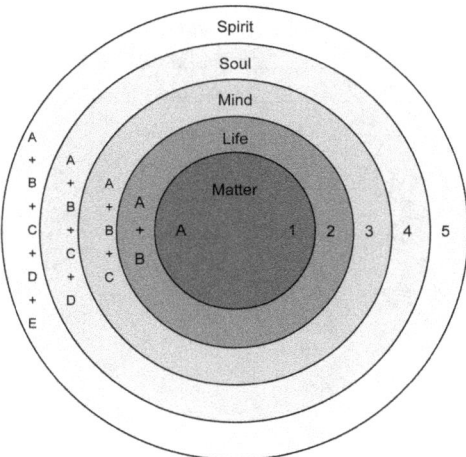

Modern, orthodox researchers have also identified the 'journey into oneself' as a universal and cross-cultural experience of multiple stages of self-identity and self-growth which we navigate by the agency of two fundamental capacities: *transcendence* and *inclusion*. First, we identify or fuse with a stage of development but, over time, as we experience events that do not conform to our existing beliefs, we are nudged to reinterpret those events, to react to them in new ways, and so we achieve more and more sophisticated levels of functional maturity. *The human mind, in sum, emerges from the interaction of the brain with*

experience. Below I offer a simplified map of the human adventure, drawing on, and extending, the work of the pre-eminent developmental psychologist, Robert Kegan (who, in turn, drew on the pioneering work of the epistemologist, Jean Piaget). Our journey begins in infancy at the *Sensorimotor* stage. There follows the *Impulsive* stage of early childhood, the *Imperial* stage of late childhood, the *Relational* stage of adolescence, and the *Organisational* stage of young adulthood, all of which most of us achieve. Only a small percentage of us achieve the subsequent *World-Centric* stage; and the highest position, the *Self-Transcendent* stage (the realm of those frontier sages and mystics), is a very rare accomplishment indeed (Cowie, 2012, pp. 13-39).

The Human Adventure

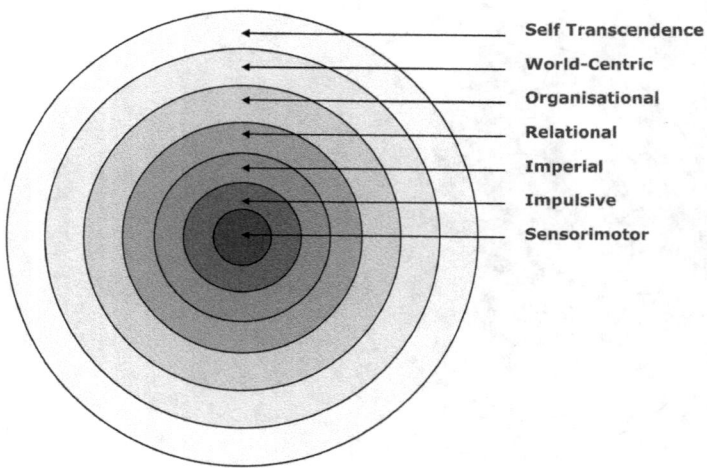

The Stages of the Human Development Journey

The Sensorimotor Stage

In the first few months of my life I cannot differentiate myself from the physical world: I am, essentially, a sensorimotor organism.

The Impulsive Stage

I am a young child now, and a separate Self with purposes of my own which I seek to fulfil. I have my own perceptions, too; and, as I cannot distinguish yet between how something appears to me and how something *is*, my life is filled with fantasy.

The Imperial Stage

As an older child, I have a self-concept and I become invested in that sense of Self through personal aggrandisement, display and competition. My care and concern extend to my group – but no further!

The Relational Stage

As an adolescent, I learn that others have needs, too, and so I become empathetic and invested in my relationships. I seek inclusion, affiliation and nurturance.

> "No individual is self-sufficient; the individual can exist only in an environmental field. The individual is inevitably, at every moment, a part of some field. His behaviour is a function of the total field, which includes both him and his environment" (Perls, 1973, pp. 15-16).

The Organisational Stage

As a young adult, I desire independence. My concern is to preserve a new-found autonomy, and to seek group recognition of it through organisational involvement.

The World-Centric Stage

At last I can embrace a truly global perspective: my group is not the only group in the universe!

The Self-Transcendent Stage

I have now achieved a depth of consciousness which is not confined to my individual Self.

The human development road may be well charted, but the journey along it is not an easy one: each stage presents a new set of challenges

– intellectual, social, moral, emotional, psychological and even spiritual challenges symbolised in those ancient stories by the fearsome creatures the Hero encounters. These challenges flow through the basic stages as developmental *streams*, and cross-cultural, empirical studies show that they unfold in the same way as the stages unfold – as clear, qualitative transformations of thinking and being, and by the same agencies of transcendence and inclusion. "We navigate this complex landscape on a spiralling pathway which integrates our achievements in all the streams, and the summation of our achievements indicates the overall stage of development that we have reached" (Cowie, 2012, pp. 43-92).

The Streams of Development

An Integral Model of Development

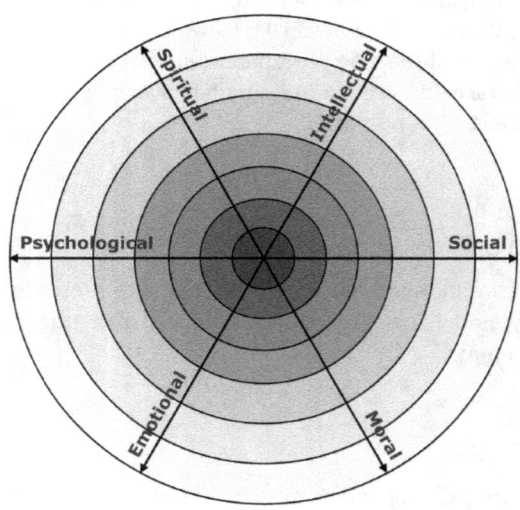

The Intellectual Stream: the process of making meaning from data – how we absorb it, organise it, interpret it, and then take action upon it. We construct our knowledge of all the domains of development by reflecting upon, and making sense of, our life experiences.

The Social Stream: the process of forging social connection, of discovering how to relate to, adapt to, and function with, other people. Our relationships are also foundational to our overall development, shaping both the structure of the brain and the emergence of the mind: the mental models of Self, and of the Self with others, that we create through our social involvements, form an 'essential scaffold' for the development of our psyche.

The Moral Stream: the process of acquiring moral reasoning – our increasingly sophisticated understanding of what is 'right' and what is 'wrong'.

The Emotional Stream: the process of learning how to manage our responses to emotionally arousing stimuli.

The Psychological Stream: the process of developing an identity – our increasingly sophisticated way of perceiving ourselves, enabling us to orientate ourselves in the world. The identity theorist, Jane Loevinger, describes identity (or the 'ego') as the central organiser (Loevinger, 1976, pp. 58-59). "Our emerging sense of who we are integrates our achievements in the other developmental domains."

The Spiritual Stream: the process of learning how to appreciate a transcendent dimension to human life.

As Robert Kegan explains, each stage of development requires its own culturing context which 'holds' us as we become embedded in it, then 'lets go' of us as we emerge from it (permitting us to explore safely to the edge of our present limits) and then 'remains in place' (enabling us to integrate all our stream-specific learning experiences into our sense of Self) as we move on to our next state of equilibrium (Kegan, 1982). "During our working lives, our organisation is our primary development context because this is where we spend most of our waking hours."

Becoming What One Is: the Firm Footing to Move

Even today, tales of quest from the distant past call us to our own adventure, but if, in our determination to press onwards, we choose not to address the full range of challenges presented to us at our current stage, we will arrive at the next stage of our journey with some of our potential unrealised, with an imbalance in our sphere of total capability. The further we travel along the pathway of growth, of course, the greater the risk of such developmental gaps appearing, and such gaps will necessarily place limitations on us as we try to manage the increasingly complex circumstances and events of our lives (Cowie, 2012, p. 44). To function *as a* "fully integrated Self", therefore, we must consolidate our position (or, in the words of Arnold Beisser, find our 'firm footing') at each stage of our development by addressing all the stream-specific learning experiences offered by our culturing context. And we must do this before we endeavour to move on to the next stage: "Change occurs when one becomes what he is, not when he tries to become what he is not" (Beisser, 1970).

Most of us, in young adulthood, achieve the Organisational stage. With a new-found autonomy we seek group recognition of it through organisational involvement: the structured and regularised culturing context of our organisational setting fosters us in our exercises of self-discipline, personal achievement, pride in ourselves and ambition. In this environment, we can find our own place; build networks of colleagues who can help us when we need them to do so; demonstrate and define ourselves through our activities; and satisfy our desire for progression, status and financial reward. Here we can fully immerse ourselves: it is the place in which we are able to be the person we have *become*.

As we consolidate our position at this stage, our 'firm footing' there is expressed as follows:

THE 'FIRM FOOTING' OF THE ORGANISATIONAL STAGE	
The Intellectual Stream	We have an increasing capacity for conceptual thinking.
The Social Stream	We construct our relationships in service of our autonomous identity.
The Moral Stream	We create a set of moral assumptions that maintains the given social order.
The Emotional Stream	We achieve independent functioning as a competent emotional being (subject, of course, to emotional hijackings from time-to-time).
The Psychological Stream	We have a heightened sense of our individuality – indeed, we define ourselves by our activities, our autonomous ways of thinking, doing and being.
The Spiritual Stream	We relocate authority from our reference group to the Self.

As with all the foregoing evolutionary stages, however, the distinguishing characteristic of the Organisational stage (its self-possession) is also its limitation. Over time, we may experience a growing sense of loneliness, even isolation in our relationships as they are currently constructed, which may be reinforced by those with whom we have them beginning to demand that we grant them their own individuality, their distinctness from the maintenance of our self-system. If we are to emerge from this developmental stage, we will need to learn to place our independent Self in the bigger context of *inter*dependence. In so doing, we will scrutinise the socio-centric perspectives in which we were previously invested as the core of our identity, and will come to recognise that our values and opinions are *not* necessarily better than those of others; they are simply different. For the first time, a Self will emerge which can embrace a truly global world-view and, if growth continues, we will move on to identify with the next stage of development, the World-Centric stage, the 'firm footing' of which is expressed as follows:

THE 'FIRM FOOTING' OF THE WORLD-CENTRIC STAGE	
The Intellectual Stream	We achieve a level of conceptual sophistication that enables us to engage in subjective, interpersonal and non-rational thought processes, and to embrace (not just manage) complexity, paradox, ambiguity, uncertainty and flux. At this level we are also able to participate in group thinking – a cognitive process which requires those involved to give up their own assumptions and opinions to allow shared meaning to emerge.
The Social Stream	We construct relationships of interdependence in which we grant others their own individuality, relationships that serve mutual needs.
The Moral Stream	Our moral assumptions embrace a universal world view.
The Emotional Stream	We continue to hone our emotional skills in what is an ongoing endeavour to manage both our positive and our negative emotions as constructively as possible.
The Psychological Stream	We have separated ourselves from our activities and have a consolidated sense of identity. Jane Loevinger believed that the highest position of this development stream is the state of 'self-actualization' which the psychologist, Abraham Maslow, researched and described. Maslow remarks of those who have reached it that they have so much to teach the rest of us that "they seem almost like a different breed of human beings" (Maslow, 1987, p. xxxv).
The Spiritual Stream	We are aware of humanity as an inclusive community of being.

There are no age-norms for the accomplishment of the World-Centric stage, and cross-cultural studies reveal that very many adults never achieve it, either because the assistance they need for their growth is not available or because they do not choose to find it. Certainly, work settings which recognise, encourage or support development beyond the Organisational stage are rare indeed – even in those enterprises that are orientated towards learning.

Collective Renewal: the Transformation of the Total Field

The Hero's 'search for Self' is not conducted solely for his own purposes: through his transformation, his community is also renewed. In Sir Thomas Malory's masterpiece of Arthurian literature, *Le Morte Darthur* (1469–1470), 150 knights of King Arthur's chivalric brotherhood, the Round Table, ride out from Camelot in search of the Grail; after many trials, Sir Percival, Sir Bors and the spiritually triumphant Sir Galahad, "the rose which ys the floure of all good vertu" (Malory, 1971, p. 600), achieve it. It is (partially) revealed to them in the Castle of Carbonek whereupon Sir Galahad is able to heal the Maimed King. The three knights then take the Grail, covered in red samite, by ship to the city of Sarras where Galahad assumes the kingship on the death of the tyrant, Estorause, "by all the assente of the hole cité" (Malory, 1971, p. 606). The marvels of the Grail are fully revealed to Sir Galahad one year later, whereupon his request to leave this earthly world is answered; Sir Perceval retires to a hermitage (to renounce all, in the Medieval monastic tradition, and pray for humankind) until *he* dies little more than a year later; and Sir Bors returns to Camelot to recount their 'hyghe adventures'. With his return, the society of the Round Table, which King Arthur worked so hard to create, is (at least temporarily) restored:

> "So aftir the quest of the Sankgreall was fulfilled and all the knyghtes that were leffte on live were com home agayne unto the Table Rownde...than was there grete joy in the courte, and enespeciall kynge Arthure and queen Gwenyvere made grete joy of the remenaunte that were com home" (Malory, 1971, p. 611).

Similarly, in our modern world, the possibility of collective renewal (for organisations and, hence, for our global community) rests on a proposition that individual development and organisation development are conjoined: if development theory holds true for individuals, then it must hold true for organisations which are, essentially, groups of such individuals operating together over a period of time in the same culture (Cowie, 2012, pp. 203–207). This is a proposition that is, of course, affirmed by General Systems Theory. As organisations are clearly intentionally-designed constructs, I would not necessarily expect them to develop *in the same way* as living organisms but I do note that, once an organisation has formed, it does exhibit some fundamental characteristics of living organisms, particularly human organisms, by striving for, for example, greater complexity, greater integration and greater differentiation in its own project of evolution, and so I do believe we can identify a sequence of developmental stages that may be applied to it. And, given the pivotal role of senior leaders in shaping it, I also believe that the mean stage of development that they, *in particular*, have reached will have a defining influence on the stage of development that the whole organisation has reached.

If, therefore, as is likely, an organisation is dominated by people at the Organisational stage (who joined it because it provides them with a venue in which they can be their autonomous selves), the prevailing holding environment will foster organisational-stage behaviour which will translate into an enterprise that *is* organisational. It will be well-structured and performance-driven. Members will rally around the corporate vision and their own tasks and targets which will have been defined for the purpose of beating or defeating the competition. "People are important" – but not at the expense of the enterprise attaining its business goals, or of it maintaining its belief-system and working principles. Investments will be made in external relationships – with other organisations and the community – but only to secure competitive advantage. Demonstrably, this is an organisation that is acting independently, *according to its own self-interest*.

Organisations today, however, are operating in the far-reaching, *interdependent* ecologies of business, society, politics, climate and the environment. They are essential elements of our shared resource-systems which are riven by man-made catastrophes such as scarcity, criminality, economic collapse, terrorism, climate-change and war, and so they are *obligated* to play their part in the necessary work of system-renewal. In the marked absence of either technical or political mechanisms for managing the commons, a new way of thinking (and therefore of being) which is not of a level of consciousness that gave rise to these multiple crises is required. This new way of thinking is, of course, the holistic, integral mode of meaning-making which is only available to us when we have reached the World Centric stage (Cowie, 2012, pp. 33–35) – when we can, for example, in our organisational lives:

- Challenge 'business as usual' and find creative solutions to problems because now we are no longer invested in the preservation of our organisation *as-it-is* as the venue in which we affirm our identity.
- Evaluate the effect that our organisation is having on the local community, the natural environment, the nation and the world because we now perceive it in the context of the wider system in which it operates.
- Propose a greater purpose for our organisation than to exist simply to maintain itself because we are now able to envision the role it *could* play in the world.
- Advocate and defend strong, self-chosen ethical principles in the exercise of our leadership because our moral perspective is now a concern for the welfare of *all* humankind.

It follows that the responsibility of Gestalt OD practitioners must be to foster the conditions that will support the development of a critical mass of colleagues who are ready to move to the World-Centric stage, so that their organisation *becomes* world-centric. As such, this organisation, will seek, coordinate and utilise the wisdom of its members to challenge, stretch and advance its purpose, its belief-system and its working principles so that it can attend to the needs of every stakeholder, and, thereby, enhance the opportunities of our interrelated and interdependent world *for all*.

System-interventions which support movement of people towards the World-Centric stage and enable them to find their 'firm footing' there

LEVEL OF SYSTEM	THE WORK OF THE GESTALT OD PRACTITIONER
At the intrapersonal level	**Be world-centric yourself!** Seize stream-specific development opportunities that will enable you to find your firm footing at this stage, and note that Abraham Maslow identified a threshold zone of 'readiness' that we must pass through *before* we can achieve 'self-actualization'. (This involves, for example, experiencing an enduring, loyal, post-romantic love relationship; shedding perfectionist illusions and becoming realistic; finding our peace with death; learning enough about evil in ourselves and others to be compassionate; and becoming post-ambivalent about parents and elders, power and authority.) We must commit to our own development if we are calling others to move forward on *their* journey of growth. And remember: role modelling world-centric behaviour does not simply 'show the way' to others; it also gives them permission to be different *from who they were* at the Organisational stage.
At the inter-individual level	**Make *meaningful* contact with the Other** • Facilitate contact between you and others in relationships of interdependence, in which you grant them their individuality, and they grant you yours. • Provide them with feedback to help them identify which world-centric challenges they have met, and which challenges they have yet to address in the different streams of development. • Help them to interpret their experiences in a world-centric context. • Help them to find solutions to the challenges they still face, as members of one community of being. • Help them to incorporate all their achievements in the different development streams, so that they can find their 'firm footing' at the World-Centric stage. • Learn from them as fellow-travellers on the human development road.

At the group level	**Help groups to do their work** • Facilitate group-development processes that enable colleagues to cease defining themselves by their own activities in order to work as a cohesive whole in which leadership is distributed. Note: it is a common misconception that organisations, as social systems, nurture team behaviour. In fact, most organisations nurture their members' individuality notwithstanding the fact that we have long known, from the study of group development that a 'high-performing team' can only emerge when autonomous ways of working have been renounced. • When complex problems arise, employ well-proven methods that have been developed to promote participatory thinking which is the medium of insight for people at the World-Centric stage: those involved rise above their own interpretations of the data, and the group mind is engaged. • Help groups (sub-systems of the whole) to map their interdependencies so that members are encouraged to give up the socio-centric stance of the Organisational stage, and create working arrangements of real connection across the enterprise.
At the Organisational Level	**Locate the system in its environment** Facilitate whole-system processes that enable the organisation to: • Expand its boundaries to 'bring the outside in', so that the outside becomes a greater and greater resource for it, and an 'opportunity' rather than an 'inconvenience' or a 'constraint'. • Envisage the role it could play in the world, and generate a purpose that is bigger than itself. • Formulate a set of values that stretches the definition of what is important to include forging relationships of mutual respect and influence. • Build a sense of identity that instils pride in members because it represents the organisation's broad perspective and commitments.

Conclusion

In *Le Morte Darthur*, the Round Table finally falls because of the failure of fellowship, the factionalism amongst the different kin groups at the Court which even King Arthur cannot resolve. Arthur's traiterous son, Mordred, usurps the crown, and mortally wounds him in the last battle before he is, himself, slain by his father. Malory's printer, William Caxton, writes in the Preface to this epic tale, "al is wryton for our doctryne" (Malory, 1971, p. xv). In Medieval Britain the threats to the commons were of a local consequence; today they are of an existential magnitude. Breakdown calls for breakthrough; system failure calls for system renewal. As practitioners of the Gestalt approach to OD, we must strive to live and work at the World-Centric stage with all the functional maturity that is available to us when we have found our 'firm footing' there as a fully integrated Self; and we must help those whom we serve to do likewise so that their organisations can become a force for good in the total field of our fragmented and individualistic, yet also interrelated and interdependent, globalised world. The 'call to adventure' is to all people of all times, but it has never been so urgent as it is today; and today it is for the many, not just the few, to answer that call.

References

Beisser, A. 'The paradoxical theory of change', *The Gestalt therapy page* [online]. Available at http://www.gestalt.org/arnie.htm.

Campbell, J. (1993) *The hero with a thousand faces.* London: Fontana Press.

Cowie, K. (2012) *Finding Merlin: a handbook for the human development journey in our new organisational world.* Singapore: Marshall Cavendish International.

Kegan, R. (1982) *The evolving self.* Cambridge, Massachusetts: Harvard University Press.

Loevinger, J. (1976) *Ego development.* San Francisco: Jossey-Bass Publishers.

Malory, Sir T. (1971) in Vinaver, E. (ed.) *The complete works.* Oxford: Oxford University Press.

Maslow, A.H. (1987) *Motivation and Personality.* 3rd edn. New York: Longman, an imprint of Addison Wesley Longman, Inc.

Perls, F. (1973) *The Gestalt approach and eye witness to therapy.* Ben Lomond, California: Science and Behavior Books, Inc.

Smuts, J.C. (1926) *Holism and evolution.* Facsimile edition. London: Forgotten Books

Von Bertalanffy, L. (1969) *General system theory: foundations, development, applications*. Revised edn. New York: George Braziller, Inc.

Wilbur, K. (2001) *A brief history of everything*. 2nd edn. Dublin: Gateway Books, an imprint of Gill and Macmillan.

Chapter 8: Gestalt Coaching for Awareness Management: The Elements of Mastery

Dorothy E. Siminovitch

A mindfulness revolution is spreading across the world in response to the fragmentation of attention caused by rapid change and disruption. The Gestalt approach, which holds awareness as core to functional well-being and new learning, is an antidote to this fragmentation. Gestalt coaching, the latest innovative application of Gestalt theory, offers coaches and their clients ways to meet 21st-century challenges of volatility, uncertainty, complexity, and ambiguity with the adaptive competencies of vision, understanding, clarity, and agility.* Gestalt coaching's theory, methods, and techniques focus on awareness processes for perceiving and responding to our world. This chapter clarifies the awareness dimensions that activate one's presence and the awareness choice points for use of self, which is the barometer of masterful coaching and leadership work.

Gestalt practice assumes that people are innately capable and competent, and have the necessary resources to manage personal and professional challenges. The pivotal requirement in Gestalt work is to facilitate clients' awareness about how they are or not satisfying their needs, wants, and goals. The power of awareness is what informs the Paradoxical Theory of Change: awareness, in itself, is a catalyst toward change and growth. As an act of intervention, heightening awareness expands clients' perceptual lenses to include more possibilities and new choices. A principal intervention is to have the client become aware of a figure of interest, the term that identifies what they are paying attention to. Figures can be clearly identifiable, or they can be obscured by too many figures or when the client is distracted by unaware resistances. Gestalt practice integrates the concept of mindfulness as "paying attention in a particular way: on purpose, in the present moment, and

---

* Bob Johansen, *Get There Early: Sensing the Future to Compete in the Present* (San Francisco: Berrett-Koehler, 2007).

nonjudgmentally."* It encourages a cognitive and emotional understanding, exploration, and investment into the awareness process as key to adaptive change and sustained learning. The power of the Gestalt approach is made visible by being experiential: what's experienced has the immediacy and retention of inside-out learning.

For example: Ted, an executive, is confronted by an employee in distress over a recent project failure. The employee's distress calls for empathy, but Ted is unable to be supportive because of his unacknowledged belief that failure is ruinous, and he resists offering empathy. If Ted were aware of his view of failure, he could examine whether that belief still holds true for him. The ability to perceive new perspectives, new opportunities of interest, or novel solutions resides in becoming aware of and managing obsolete resistances. Rather than acting as a "self-aware" leader who has "emotional intelligence," Ted, being unaware of the depths of his own fear of failure, lacked the relevant emotional skills to respond to his employee. His unawareness has broader impact: self-aware leaders are found to be adept and effective at both engaging their employees and achieving bottom-line results.†

Effective Gestalt coaching will trigger unaware resistances, requiring clients' willingness to risk being vulnerable in the service of new learning and new skills. The coach's presence is a critical resource supporting clients to confront their discomfort. Ted's fear of failure suggests a benefit from coaching to understand how he has alienated his capacity to show compassion for those experiencing failure. Coaching can give him a safe place to explore his lack of empathy around this issue, and to experiment with ways he might offer more emotionally appropriate responses, both to himself and others. The Gestalt coach, using her own presence, would encourage Ted's work by expressing her understanding of his fear of failure and demonstrating her compassion for his difficulties.

---

* Jon Kabat-Zinn, *Wherever You Go, There You Are: Mindfulness Meditation in Everyday Life* (New York: Hyperion, 1994), 4.

† J. P. Flaum, "When It Comes to Business Leadership, Nice Guys Finish First," Green Peak Partners, 2010. The study was conducted in association with Cornell University's School of Industrial and Labor Relations. Retrieved from http://greenpeakpartners.com/uploads/Green-Peak_Cornell-University-Study_What-predicts-success.pdf. Kevin Cashman, "Return on Self-Awareness: Research Validates the Bottom Line of Leadership Development," *Forbes* March 17, 2014. Retrieved from https://www.forbes.com/sites/kevincashman/2014/03/17/return-on-self-awareness-research-validates-the-bottom-line-of-leadership-development/#197a68363750.

Presence and Use of Self

Gestalt coaching is driven by practitioner competency in understanding and applying two core concepts: *Presence* and *Use of Self*. Presence is the embodiment and incubator of one's essential identity. Use of self is the intentional leveraging of one's presence to influence outcomes related to needs and goals, one's own or others'. We manifest our presence through exchange, which reveals our values, mindsets, and style or aesthetics. As coaches or leaders, we can think of presence as a *being* intervention: simply "showing up" has an evocative effect, the first indication of whether or how people will work with us. Though we may not be able to predict how our presence will affect others, we are responsible for the self-work of reflection and asking to learn what we evoke in others.

Use of self is a *doing* intervention: the purposeful actions we take with others to provoke their movement toward greater awareness and defined goals. Use of self is a practitioner competency where we consciously exercise the dimensions of our presence to provoke action toward attaining what is needed, wanted, or missing. One integrative task of developing one's presence and use of self in Gestalt coaching is attending to and being aligned with one's personal strengths, values, and intentions for influence. Authenticity is increased by this alignment. As presence is only relationally experienced, coaches and leaders alike have to manage their Perceived Weirdness Index (PWI), which refers to our perceived degree of "difference" relative to others.[*] This means knowing how to strategically relate to others with enough similarity so that they feel the comfort of familiarity, but also with enough difference so that they are interested in working with us. If our differences are greater than the value we bring to the work, the PWI may be too high to serve the coach or leader. Awareness of our PWI necessarily invites us to be more alert and adaptive, offering similarity as an interpersonal bridge and unique perspectives and skills as a differential value.

---

[*] Mary Ann Rainey Tolbert and Jonno Hanafin, "Use of Self in OD Consulting: What Matters Is Presence," pp. 78–79. In *The NTL Handbook of Organization Change and Development: Principles, Practices, and Perspectives*, edited by Brenda B. Jones and Michael Brazzel (San Francisco: Pfeiffer, 2006).

Presence Awareness Dimensions

Presence has extensive expression across individuals, but can be described through a seven-dimension structure which captures the requisite variety to meet contemporary life and work challenges.[*] The dimensions can be developed to respond to and manage the range of awarenesses needed for coaches and leaders. These dimensions are: self-aware alignment with and embodiment of one's values; creativity; emotions and emotional range; capacity for heart-based or caring relations; communication and voice; intuition; and scanning the field for threats and opportunities.[†] Each dimension of presence is positively defined by what we pay attention to, and limited by unaware resistances that interfere or stop us from being aware of that dimension and acting in congruence with our values and with related dimensions. Our presence can be strengthened or weakened by intentional practices of our use of self. We can strengthen our presence through self-work in each dimension to guide our use of self skills. We can assess our use of self skills by inviting feedback and observations about our interventions, projections about how people are experiencing our actions, and inquiry regarding our impact. (Figure 1.1) Inviting this kind of information is a commitment towards mastery.

---

[*] The term "requisite variety" comes from Ross Ashby, a cyberneticist and psychiatrist. The most applicable definition for our purposes is that someone can only model or control something to the extent that she herself has sufficient internal variety to represent it. F. Heylighen and C. Joslyn, "The Law of Requisite Variety," August 31, 2001. Retrieved from http://pespmc1.vub.ac.be/REQVAR.html.

[†] Dorothy E. Siminovitch, *A Gestalt Primer: The Path Toward Awareness IQ* (2017), pp. 110-125.

Figure 1.1 Awareness Dimensions and Choice Points

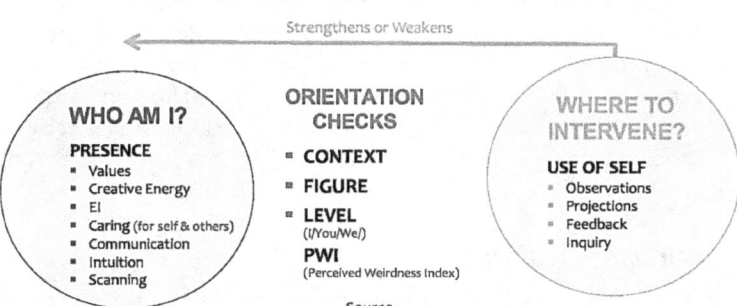

Dimension 1: Self-Aware Alignment with Embodied Values

Understanding and knowing yourself means knowing your values and beliefs, and knowing when you've been derailed from your core identity. Your values, and the clarity and consistency with which you communicate those, somatically or verbally, are seen by others as signaling trustworthiness. A 2016 Harvard Business School survey of leadership learning and development programs reveals that "demonstrating integrity" is the top-ranked leadership capability.[*] The demonstration of one's values through consistent language and behavior is perceived by others as authentic and inspiring. When volatility, uncertainty, complexity, and ambiguity arise, we are supported by our aware values and goals, and we learn how to return to our core identity when we're thrown off course. Self-awareness entails tracking your sensations, thoughts, emotions, resistances, and mindsets to keep them aligned with your identity during disruption. Gestalt coaches understand how to track values, how to identify resistances that derail clients, and how to offer practices to manage them. (Figure 1.2)

---

[*] Harvard Business School Corporate Learning, "The State of Leadership Development," 2016. Retrieved from https://www.harvardbusiness.org/sites/default/files/19770_CL_StateOfLeadership_Report_July2016.pdf. "Demonstrating Integrity" was closely followed by: managing complexity, inspiring engagement, and acting strategically.

Figure 1.2 Self-Aware Alignment with Embodied Values

VALUE	UNAWARE RESISTANCES	SUGGESTED PRACTICES
• Sense of purpose • Energy for taking action • Inspiring trust and commitment	• Need to feel unique • Outdated "shoulds" • Fear of identity challenges	• Be transparent – share your vision, values, and goals • Ask for feedback – invite connection

Dimension 2: Creativity

Creativity calls upon the desire for novelty and opens opportunities to discover new possibilities. Creativity includes being open to using the knowledge and expertise of others as well as gathering ideas from diverse sources. The way we support, demonstrate, and communicate creativity affects how others perceive and receive innovative ideas and different ways of doing things. (Figure 1.3)

Figure 1.3 Creativity

VALUE	UNAWARE RESISTANCES	SUGGESTED PRACTICES
• Outwitting obsolescence • Gaining a broad range of diverse ideas for innovative solutions • Energizing others' engagement with challenges	• Fear of failure • Shame of being "mediocre" • Losing managerial control of the process	• Reflecting on failure for learning and growth • Inviting early failure • Inviting feedback

Dimension 3: Emotions and Emotional Range

Emotional Intelligence (EI) refers to the ability to recognize, understand, and manage one's own emotions, while also being able to recognize, understand, and influence the emotions of others. EI means being aware of your current emotional state and the emotional triggers that might derail you. When you can name your emotions, make meaning from what you're feeling, and exercise emotional self-regulation, you have the essential relational skills which strengthen presence and use of self. Self-reflection and feedback help us understand whether our emotions are supporting or limiting us. Emotions are a "gut" gauge for what really matters. Important matters typically arouse excitement or anxiety. If no emotional energy is present, the idea or activity may not have enough interest to merit investment. If strong emotions are present but disregarded, you may later have to manage the unfinished business of regret or dissatisfaction. (Figure 1.4)

Figure 1.4 Emotions and Emotional Range

VALUE	UNAWARE RESISTANCES	SUGGESTED PRACTICES
• Knowing what matters to you and to others • Emotional dexterity in responding to others • Being able to regulate the emotions involved, and thereby create safety and trust	• Distrusting the value of emotions • Perceiving emotions as disturbances rather than information • Seeing emotional vulnerability as a sign of weakness	• Develop a habit of naming strong emotions and pausing before reacting. With practice, greater choice becomes available. • Mindful breathing is helpful: Inhale for 4 seconds, exhale for 5 seconds. After 5 such breaths, a relaxation response is stimulated. With practice, you'll feel a shift to calm awareness after just a few such deep breaths.

Dimension 4: Heart-Based or Caring Relations

The capacity to care about others is an essential human attribute. Leaders who convey a sense of caring about the well-being of their employees and colleagues establish resonance: "a powerful, positive emotional reality . . . that is marked by hope, enthusiasm and the collective will to win. Resonance makes people feel good: committed, willing to work hard, and passionate about results."* Heart-based relationships call for the vulnerability of intimacy, the capacity to forgive and move forward, and the willingness to form relationships without strategic agendas. Leaders must learn to be mindful and caring about their own well-being while also caring about and connecting with others. (Figure 1.5)

Figure 1.5 Heart-Based Relations

VALUE	UNAWARE RESISTANCES	SUGGESTED PRACTICES
• Engaging with self and others in ways that motivate and inspire • Strengthening cross-organizational relationships • Energizing optimism and hope	• Being rejected • Being taken advantage of • Losing positional control • Identity diffusion or confusion (losing personal boundaries)	• Give positive affirmations, to self and others, and show appreciation frequently • Establish relationships across departmental and division boundaries that are non-strategic

Dimension 5: Communication and Voice

Communication is a purposeful activity to express and share an idea, information, or collective vision. The exchange intends to inform, motivate, or inspire. Accuracy and transparency are figural attributes of trusted communication. If a message has changed due to unexpected issues, people need to be informed, especially if what has changed contradicts what was previously communicated. In professional venues, we may need to change our minds based on new information, but we must be able and willing to explain why the change was necessary. (Figure 1.6)

---

* Annie McKee and Abhijit Bhaduri, "Resonant Leadership for Results," Teleos Leaders June 3, 2013. Retrieved from http://www.teleosleaders.com/2013/06/03/resonant-leadership-for-results/.

Figure 1.6 Communication and Voice

VALUE	UNAWARE RESISTANCES	SUGGESTED PRACTICES
• Increased trust, engagement, and commitment • Providing common ground for crucial decision-making processes • Encouraging participatory, creative problem-solving	• Fear of being seen as incompetent • Loss of control • Loss of being the one to turn to for information and guidance	• Inquire: *Ask* people what they want or need to know • Ask for feedback about how your communications are working or not working to achieve your intent • Incorporate the Speech Acts: Declarations, Assessments, Assertions, Promises, and Requests[*]

Dimension 6: Intuition

Intuition's ancient attraction has resurfaced in today's leadership literature as a valued resource, especially in conditions of uncertainty and ambiguity when data is scarce or unavailable but a quick response is needed. An intuitive answer seems to come effortlessly, in a flash, but studies suggest it's a recognition of patterns discerned from accumulated experiential and cognitive knowledge. Given the right confluence of circumstances and awareness practices, intuition offers valid solutions in moments of uncertainty. However, it's important to differentiate intuition from an unaware agenda, e.g., an emotional reaction tied to some past event or personal issue. (Figure 1.7)

---

[*] Chalmers Brothers, *Language and the Pursuit of Happiness: A New Foundation for Designing Your Life, Your Relationships, and Your Results* (Naples, FL: New Possibilities Press, 2005), p. 154.

Figure 1.7 Intuition

VALUE	UNAWARE RESISTANCES	SUGGESTED PRACTICES
• A strong resource when accurately tracked and verified • Gives us initial "heart" and "gut" conceptions of a person or situation that can be useful in guiding our interactions	• Being thought of as weird • Being socially isolated • Being wrong	• Allow for self-reflection time and/or short meditations that make intuition more available • Share your intuitions with trusted others and ask for feedback • Manage your Perceived Weirdness Index (PWI)

Dimension 7: Scanning the Field for Threats and Opportunities

Scanning means watching for what's emerging on the horizon of possibility as an opportunity or threat. To be effective, credible, and inspiring, leaders have to see the "big picture," and to take some risks in naming what they see emerging. When they spot an opportunity or threat, they put their own values on the line to advocate an action or policy that they believe aligns with the organization's mission and the employees' collective values in order to build mutual advantage in their immediate and extended business communities. (Figure 1.8)

Figure 1.8 Scanning the Field

VALUE	UNAWARE RESISTANCES	SUGGESTED PRACTICES
• Differentiating between a threat and an opportunity • Recognizing an opportunity in what appears to be a threat • Recognizing the implicit threat in an opportunity	• Being in a state of uncertainty or ambiguity • Not having the data that offers control of the situation • Being wrong or incompetent	• Ask for input and engage in discussion with your teams and peers • Attend major professional conferences and engage in thought activities that give you up-to-date information and insights about your field

Orientation Checks and Process Tools for Intervention Mastery

The seven outlined dimensions of presence awareness are inner resources for coaches and leaders to access. The orientation checks are what activate the interplay between the dimensions of presence and use of self (see Figure 1.1). Context (e.g., purpose, environment or setting, people involved) is critical to determine what is expected or outside the norms, and is a broader expression of PWI management. The Gestalt coach seeks the figure, like Ted's fear of failure, which has the most interest or energy for the client. Awareness of the figure is needed to better organize observations, aware projections, feedback, and inquiry. After identifying the figure, it is important to determine which level of system (LOS) holds the work—individual, interpersonal, or group. The Cycle of Experience (COE) is a tool to determine both the figure and the boundary of the work to manage and prevent incorrect LOS awareness, thus allowing focus on the appropriate intervention process.

Process Tools

Gestalt coaching gives leaders experiential opportunities to explore how they "show up" to others and to experiment with how to use themselves effectively. It is the Cycle of Experience with the Unit of Work (UOW) that are process tools that aid the coach's shaping of these opportunities.* The COE is a tool to track awareness moments and the habitual patterns that serve or interfere with goal attainment. Using the COE with our executive Ted allowed him to become aware of his sensations of discomfort and shame around offering sympathy in relation to failure. Using the COE, the coach can gauge when to offer observations, make projections, and give data-based feedback. The COE made figural to Ted that he managed his discomfort and shame by avoiding situations that were in fact opportunities to offer compassion and support around failure.

The UOW is a process structure designed to explore an important issue revealed by the COE that's of interest to the client. UOW invitations

---

* The COE and the UOW are discussed in detail in *A Gestalt Coaching Primer: The Path Toward Awareness IQ* (2017): Chapter 3 (pp. 55-80) and Chapter 6 (143-166), respectively.

reveal the Gestalt coach's mastery through their use of self to support the client's awareness and action around what is needed, wanted, or missing. Ted, who couldn't offer compassion to his distressed employee, failed a critical leadership opportunity to engage his employee in a heart-based interaction rooted in emotional intelligence. If the coach perceives Ted to be poorly aligned with his value around supporting his employees, he could be offered experimental situations in which to better identify, articulate, and inhabit his core values. Ted's emotional resistance to expressing compassion might involve a breathing exercise or a dream experiment to bring him into closer contact with his emotions. If Ted expresses being "stuck" around the issue of failure, the coach could design experiments involving emotional expression and other creative modalities. If Ted is anxious about the uncertainties of failure, he could be invited to remember and reflect on past experiences when his intuitive or emotional understanding supported his ability to move forward. If Ted feels misunderstood by his employees, the coach can work to clarify how his body language and vocabulary contribute to his "message." The Gestalt coach can collaboratively design experiments where Ted can safely explore his fear of failure with self-compassion, as well as experiment with small steps by which he could build his ability to express empathy. The learning for Ted would be to reassess how the practice of giving emotional support could make him a stronger leader. Ted's case illustrates how Gestalt coaches highlight and use awareness opportunities so that clients can experientially grasp how their unaware and/or outdated beliefs are limiting their leadership.

The COE and UOW process tools offer Gestalt coaches opportunities to work with client awareness and strategically offer observations, aware projections, data-based feedback, and transformative inquiry. These interventions stimulate unexpected discoveries and alternative choices that open pathways to new behaviors, outcomes that illustrate the liberating quality of Gestalt coaching and Gestalt practice, for coaches and particularly for clients. Learning and growth are influenced by the degree of self-awareness and the use of one's awareness. If a situation calls for the leader to affirm and stand for their values, can they? If a situation calls for creativity, can the leader invite the conditions for sharing new ideas? If there is emotional intensity, can the leader manage the emotions? If an employee appears stressed and care is called for, can the leader offer the needed empathy and compassion? If important information or ideas need to be shared, can the leader communicate these at the right time in the right ways? If an issue is unclear and data unavailable, can the leader call upon intuition to offer an inspiring insight or solution? If the future seems threatening, can the leader point to emerging possibilities that offer opportunity?

Why Gestalt? Why Now?

Leaders are under increasing pressure to deliver exceptional outcomes, in employee engagement and retention and in bottom-line results. Gestalt coaching is the leadership coaching approach which most effectively addresses and cultivates the qualities defined in today's leadership literature as being most desired: leaders' ability to identify, enhance, and activate their personal values, particular strengths, and multiple resources to support their employees and benefit the organization's mission and goals. Frederick Buechner suggests that what you feel "right" in doing is perhaps what everyone needs you to be doing, right now.*

In this fast-paced world, existing knowledge may not keep pace with emergent disruptions. Mindful multi-dimensional awareness can be accessed to support perceptions of new possibilities and choices. Responding to challenges by being self-aware and using one's self strategically is a sign of mastery that inspires both coaches and their leadership clients. Gestalt awareness practices empower us to develop dimensions of our presence in alignment with our core values and to use ourselves with the intention to respond to and influence others adaptively. Being self-aware, using orientation checks and process tools to identify obstructive patterns and figures of interest, and to then use our awareness to act in the world with clarity and purpose is the mastery now called for. The skills and techniques of awareness management seem invisible until masterful practice reveals them to be vital competencies. Gestalt coaching shows how these core awareness skills and techniques can be taught, practiced, and made visibly powerful. For Gestalt coaches and for their leadership clients, self-awareness and strategic use of self are experienced as illumination and transformation.

---

* Ryan Pemberton, "Frederick Buechner on Calling: Your Deep Gladness and the World's Deep Hunger," *Called: My Journey to C. S. Lewis's House and Back Again* December 22, 2014. Buechner's exact quote is: "The place God calls you to is the place where your deep gladness and the world's deep hunger meet." Retrieved from http://www.calledthejourney.com/blog/2014/12/17/frederick-buechner-on-calling.

If our presence strongly embodies our values and best intentions, our presence alone may be enough to make a difference: people may feel calmed or supported or inspired just by being in our presence. Whether in coaching or in the workplace, though, we need to use strategic use of self practices to accomplish specific goals. Gestalt coaching interventions are organic, relevant, resonant, and uniquely suited to give today's leaders the support and practices for the vision, understanding, clarity, and agility necessary today. Coaches and leaders need to respond from a self-aware, embodied presence and with a masterful use of self to spur learning and opportunity.

Chapter 9: The Executive's Gestalt

Ollie Malone, Jr.

There can be no question as to the relevance and essential nature of leadership in organizations today. Whether the organization is a small one, a large one, or one that is being managed out of the owner's garage, leadership is an essential element. In this chapter, we will consider the role of the executive: what it is and how it can be done better. It is my hope that readers will see their own leadership and that of others more clearly and, further, that readers will also be able to see others' leadership more clearly. The ability to see these leadership elements more clearly should enable greater intervention – whether in one's own work, or in the work of others, that will, ideally, create better outcomes.

Although individuals show up in the world as whole beings – and not a collection of mis-matched parts, the functioning of individuals often lacks a sense of cohesion. Put another way, most organizations require their employees to be at least 16 years of age in order to work there, yet individuals' behaviors, actions, and reactions, may fall short of that chronological limbo stick. Over the course of the pages of this chapter, I would like to explore:
- An expanded application of the term "executive" and the implications of the use of that term for a broader audience;
- The contributions of the notion of a "Gestalt" and the insights available to us who would form an "executive Gestalt;"
- Exploration of the ways in which the "executive Gestalt" impacts ways of being in organizations and in life, in general;
- Three key directional sections of this chapter relate to Awakening the Executive's Gestalt, where the executive expands his or her awareness to include ways of thinking and being that may be new or unproven; Accelerating the Executive's Gestalt, where this new way of being becomes regularly and consistently chosen – with increasingly more attractive outcomes; and Expanding the Executive's Gestalt, where the work of the executive is to stimulate expanded awareness on the part of others within his or her universe.

Fundamental Concepts

At the outset, it may be important to clarify the use of the term "executive." Some will assume that, by the use of the term, we refer to those who are at the top rung of the organization's structure. That is not the meaning that is employed in this chapter.

The meaning assumed here aligns with Peter Drucker's in his classic work, *The Effective Executive*:

What is an executive? Every knowledge worker in modern organizations is an "executive" if, by virtue of his [or her] position or knowledge, he [or she] is responsible for a contribution that materially affects the capacity of the organization to perform and to obtain results. This may be the capacity of a business to bring out a new product or to obtain a larger share of a given market. It may be the capacity of a hospital to provide beside care to its patients, and so on. Such a man (or woman) must make decisions; he [or she] cannot just carry out orders. He [or she] must take responsibility for his [or her] contribution. And he [or she] is supposed, by virtue of his [or her] knowledge, to be better equipped to make the right decisions than anyone else. He [or she] may be overridden; he [or she] may be demoted or fired. But as long as he [or she] has the job the goals, the standards, and the contribution are in his [or her] keeping. (pp. 5-6)

The increasing complexity of the world we live and operate in has created a significant challenge for those who would be leaders:
- He or she can focus on areas of immediate concern (i.e., my salary, my team, my company, my customers, etc.) creating a leadership universe that is largely self-satisfying, but likely to leave other feeling like pawns, indentured servants, or disposable tools. For example, Edwin:
    - Edwin's last role was an international one. He had packed up his large family, all his earthly goods, and moved to an international location that he thought would create fame and fortune for him. When he was asked to leave that role, he knew his best option was to return to America. Having moved back to the United States, he was not able to find a position of similar remuneration and, as a result, had to accept a salary that was approximately 30 percent less than he had been paid before – not including a generous annual bonus. Despite this, he was confident that he could make an impact in the smaller, less-demanding organization that he

had joined. His initial energies were spent on getting the biggest salary he could negotiate and, when he had tapped out that source, finding ways that he could "beef up" his compensation. Those around him soon learn that their greatest value was the degree to which they could identify creative compensation, recognition, or reward strategies – that would benefit Edwin.

- She or he can focus on areas of longer-termed concern (i.e., the five years of the strategic plan, strategic leadership planning, long-term leadership development, the companies we'd like to acquire in the next five years) creating an audience of big-picture thinkers, yet unable to resolve the most immediate problems and concerns;
    - When Mary took over the multinational firm for which she had worked since college, she knew what her focus needed to be: to help her organization see a future that had not been considered, planned for, nor influenced. Her primary energies were spent in shifting the organization's energy to the future and she accomplished this through workshops, seminars, speeches by futurists, and intentional shifts of her time and attention to the future – often to the exclusion of other concerns.
- He or she could advance the "random" or "chaos" disciplines of leadership where, like a pinball in a pinball machine, he or she bounces off of unpredictable items with unpredictable responses – leaving those around them frustrated, perplexed, and largely wishing they were somewhere other than this unfocused, undisciplined leadership.
    - Doug was both thrilled and shocked to discover that he was the candidate selected to lead this well-established business. Although he built a strong case for himself, he could not have imagined, in his wildest dreams, that the organization's board would have selected him for its top role. Having moved into this unexpected role, he found himself at a loss as to what to do first. His instincts suggested to him that a worthy direction would be for him to work at pleasing those who had put him in position. Taking cues, then, from the verbal and nonverbal statements provided by the board, Doug used these datapoints to create his leadership agenda. Since the board was seldom of one mind (on anything), Doug found himself ricocheting from idea to idea, initiative to initiative, and

grand idea to grand idea – often contradicting work he had championed days or weeks early. Those around him found him dizzying, frustrating, and unworthy of their best efforts. Turnover became a regular and unfortunate occurrence.
- She or he could choose a more thoughtful, mindful, and eyes-on-the-prize approach to the leadership challenge being faced. This approach requires the integration of all the executive's resources and the intentional consideration of the "who, what, when, where, why, and how" of the engagement of those resources to produce the desired outcomes. It is a higher order of functioning and requires years, if not decades, of dedicated practice. Consider the story of Robin:
  - After more than 25 years of dedicated, innovative service, Robin was able to ascend the corporate ladder to the top rung at WKT, Inc. This multinational firm had observed Robin's growth and development in countless roles held: as a management trainee, as an account manager on one of the company's most difficult accounts, as a zone manager, regional manager, entrepreneurial project leader on one of the company's most successful start-ups, and in a variety of corporate assignments (supply chain, human resources, operations, and others). Along the way, Robin had amassed a strong reputation as a "company woman," a "leader of leaders" and one who clearly had a bright future ahead of her. WKT had fended off countless attempts by other organizations to lure Robin away. She had remained faithful to the organization who hired her as a trainee fresh out of college and the organization remained faithful to her. After ascending the corporate ladder, celebrating with friends and family, and settling in to her new responsibilities, Robin began to feel more exhausted than usual. It was easy for her to blame her exhaustion on the physical toll of the transition into the new role, but it seemed to be more than that. After some back-and-forth with her family on the most appropriate thing to do, Robin finally saw her physician. Then came the diagnosis: Stage 3 ovarian cancer.

Each of the categories identified above and the situations that provided additional explanation on the phenomenon occurring help to underscore the criticality of what is called in this chapter as the "Executive Gestalt." The ability to understand and work with this Executive Gestalt will make the difference between a highly effective executive and one who significantly misses the mark in his or her performance.

Figure 1: The executive and the environment are intertwined.

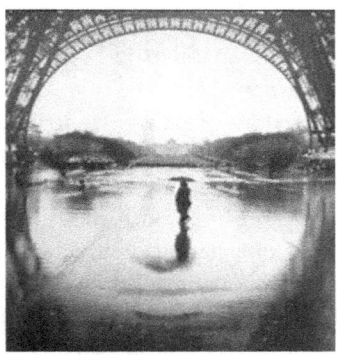

What is "The Executive's Gestalt?"

Medical professionals, psychologists, and those familiar with the workings of the human brain know that there is a set of functions within the brain that are known as "executive functions." These functions are not relegated to high-ranking leaders only, but rather refer to the higher-order part of the brain that brings some of the brain's most critical functions together for the best possible human functioning. Within the context of brain functions, "executive function" refers to the ability to:

- Manage time;
- Pay attention;
- Switch focus;
- Plan and organize;
- Remember details;
- Avoid saying or doing the wrong thing;
- Do things based on your experience;
- Multitask.

A review of this list should reveal that these functions are not unique to executives alone. Every individual needs a healthy dosage of these skills to manage her or his life. The absence of these skills produces several learning challenges in children and, in adults, produces performance challenges that, apart from intervention, can create life functioning challenges.

The "Gestalt" addition to the phrase, "The Executive's Gestalt" comes from the word "Gestalt," meaning "whole." The power in the word

"Gestalt" comes from the well-used phrase, "The whole is greater than the sum of its parts." In this manner, the phrase "The Executive's Gestalt" is used to mean:

1. The willingness to scan the major "systems" over which the executive has responsibility. The term "systems" is used to mean structures, collections of activities, and interactions that have an impact on the organization's ability to achieve its results;
2. The ability to see parts **and** wholes, hence, the ability to not only see the "systems" reference above in isolation, but to see these systems as they interact with other systems since it is often in the interaction (or lack thereof) that the organization achieves victory or defeat;
3. The ability to notice elements, to quickly sort and select those elements that are relevant and to separate them from those elements that are irrelevant;
4. The ability to notice what is NOT being noticed, to provide ample focus on the unnoticed phenomenon and to decide as to whether notice needs to shift.
5. The ability to appropriately shift focus when new information emerges requiring such a shift;
6. The ability to integrate relevant data appropriately to determine the planning and organizing that needs to occur. This does not require the complete planning and complete analysis of all that needs to be done, but the major headlines and milestones around which the remainder of the planning and analysis work should be organized.
7. The ability to capture relevant information about the organization's functioning in such a way that the information can be useful in current or future decision making. Although the "capturing" may be in the executive's head, it is usually most valuable if the capturing is done in a way that makes the information acquired accessible to others who may also be in decision-making roles.
8. The executive's ability to access relevant information that may be within his or her own experience and a potentially valuable treasure trove of information, tools, approaches, and insights. This information could be facts, intuitive beliefs, assumptions, or "gut checks" or some combination of the above. All too often, the intuitive beliefs that the executive possesses may be dismissed as being too "soft headed." It is the author's contention that the value of intuitive information lies in the executive's ability to unpack this information – either through

CHAPTER 9: THE EXECUTIVE'S GESTALT

his or her own efforts, or with the help of a coach, colleague, or consultant, so that the complex web of intuitive data can be seen, understood and appreciated by others in decision-making roles.

9   The ability to recognize the presence or absence of energy in the organization. Ultimately, the organization grows or dies because of organizational energy. Although others may frame the "energy" phenomenon using different words, fundamentally the presence of positive energy propels the organization forward. The presence of negative energy typically hovers over an organization like a wet, nasty blanket that remained in the nearby swamp overnight.

10 The ability to say the right things and encourage others to say the right things – statements that stimulate positive organizational energy, breakthrough, or an additional perspective on the challenges that might lie before individuals, teams, or an entire organization. Some of the right things useful to enhancing organization energy include:
    - Public praise and celebrations for completed tasks;
    - Public recognition of those whose extraordinary efforts made a difference in the organization's outcomes;
    - Public recognition of those in other departments whose teamwork and commitment benefit multiple parts of the organization's desired outcomes.
    - Visual displays (i.e., scoreboards) reflecting organizational progress toward goals;
    - Publication of successes achieved in print and video communication tools providing recognition of those whose efforts were central to the success achieved.

11 The ability to avoid saying the wrong things in the organization and to monitor the actions of others to ensure that they do not say the wrong things. These "wrong things" can be defined as statements that distract the organization from its primary purpose or tasks. Common distractions in most organizations include:
    - Dysfunctional gossip;
    - Internal backbiting
    - Turf wars
    - Public criticism
    - Screaming, yelling that exposes other uninvolved groups to the public derision being expressed toward team members.

12 The ability to maintain a view on multiple actions occurring in

the organization. Much like the individual on the old Ed Sullivan Show, the executive must keep several plates spinning on the end of sticks without letting any of the plates fall.

13 The ability to take care of oneself while also taking care of those in strongest connection. This requires the executive to be in tune with his or her own needs as well as the needs of family or other intimate systems. All too often, it is believed that the executive must sacrifice him or herself in service to the organization. This, we believe, is not a cause for celebration; it is martyrdom and martyrdom that will not result in a statue being erected in the executive's honor. He or she will simply be replaced with the next victim of unbridled self-sacrifice.

14 Develop and maintain healthy, functional relationships within multiple spheres of influence: one's family and intimate systems, personal and professional networks of which the executive is a member, work colleagues whose involvement and partnership is key to the desired outcomes of the work being undertaken, appropriate relationships with colleagues, clients, customers and other key work-related interpersonal relationships.

15 The ability to hold all of these dimensions named in proper and dynamic relationship – recognizing needed shifts in focus, attention, and intensity based on the needs of the environment, the needs of the various dimensions, and the executive's own values, goals, and vision.

These fifteen dimensions allow the executive to not only attend to the needs of the various systems of which she or he is a part, but also attend to her or his inner workings – the governing processes that create awareness of the other systems as well as the relative importance of those systems at any given time.

Anderson and Adams, in *Mastering Leadership* (2016), share this notion of effective leadership as a whole, not a collection of disparate parts. Their model further details the parts and, through that model, helps to identify where gaps and dysfunction may be observed.

Who cares About the Executive's Gestalt?

This expanded view of reality, or Gestalt, equips the alert executive in a number of ways. Through it, the executive sees what he or she may have previously overlooked. It is as if he or she can now see in full color that which was only previously available in muted grays.

Figure 2: Seeing oneself is central to the executive's Gestalt.

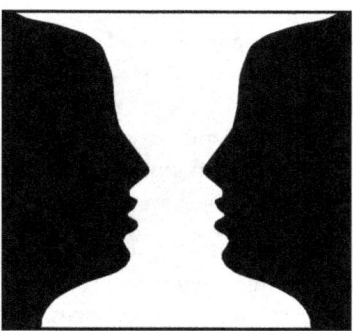

A well-developed executive Gestalt should enable the executive to:
1. See his/her own behavior clearly as well as understand the impact of his or her behavior on others with whom one works;
2. Process the impact of his or her actions cognitively (through the head), emotionally (through the heart) and primally (through the gut). Given the fact that hearers of the executive's words will be understanding them through one of these domains, the ability to flex into and out of these domains will be of infinite value in predicting the impact of one's actions as well as the ability to gain feedback on one's actions *in the moment* – allowing for far quicker response and self-correction that would have been previously available.
3. Engage with others more fully – based on the ability to access greater empathy in interpersonal interactions as well as the ability to make sense of these interactions in ways that reflect and support the needs of other parties in the interaction.
4. Function at larger and larger levels of system (interactional complexity: beginning with one-on-one interactions, small group interactions, larger group interactions, and increasingly greater levels interactions up to and including companies and even societies). The functioning at a variety of levels of system should also enable the executive to shuttle between the levels of system where it may be necessary. Imagine, for example, that I might be having a conversation with my administrative assistant. In order to understanding the depth and complexity

of that interaction, it might be useful for me to consider several interactions that may be occurring at that moment:
- The interaction of a man to a woman;
- The interaction of an African-American man to a white woman;
- The interaction of a member of our organization's "senior staff" with a member of the organization's administrative staff;
- The interaction of someone who was born and raised in a large U.S. city with someone who was born and raised in a country outside of the United States.

To the degree that the executive can expand his or her Gestalt, the executive is more able to effectively interact with individuals and groups from a variety of settings and circumstances. The executive's effectiveness, then, is highly dependent upon her or his ability to comprehend the multiple factors at play in what may seem like a relatively simplistic interaction. There is more reality available than meets the untrained eye; having effectively awakened this latent Gestalt capability, the executive is far better able to access rich information which would, otherwise, be unavailable. But how does the executive begin the process of awakening this Gestalt? The following chapters should provide useful insight.

Awakening the Executive's Gestalt

In order for the executive to fully engage his or her Gestalt, he or she must spend time stimulating a greater understanding of what this Gestalt it and how it is currently operating in his life's realities. The author is in the process of creating a journal for the sole purpose of developing a deeper awareness of the current functioning of The Executive's Gestalt and what the executive might want to do in order to create different outcomes from the information he or she may acquire through this new-found awareness. The author's contact information is available at the end of this chapter through which interested parties can acquire some of the tools that are being developed to increase the executive's ability to manage the many systems that are a part of his or her universe.

Figure 3: Accessing that which might be invisible emerges as a function of focused awareness.

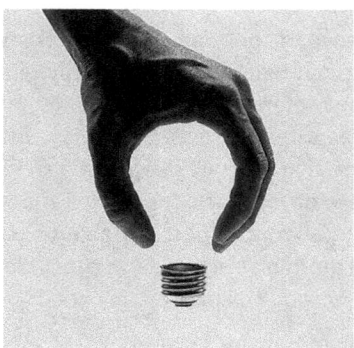

The greatest tool that the executive has to enable his or her Gestalt is the tool of **awareness.** Imagine for a moment that you have been traveling from your home or office to a destination that is unfamiliar to you. Having taken the taxi or rental car from the airport, you stumble into the hotel, provide your credit card and form of payment, grab a key and head to the room that will be your domicile for the evening.

Because you are absolutely exhausted from the day's work and travel, you quickly get out of your clothes and violently toss yourself at the bed, beginning what you expect will be a long, uninterrupted night's sleep. Ahhhh.

Several hours later, however, you are awakened by that pesky bladder of yours that is serving to remind you that you need to find your way to the bathroom, lest you create a very embarrassing situation for yourself in this heavenly bed you've been occupying.

Since you were so exhausted, however, you don't fully recall where lamp was. You assume that it's in reasonably close proximity to the bed (since that's where most hotels put them), you carefully feel around the bed, finding the night stand, then feel around the nightstand until you find the long-awaited lamp. You continue feeling around the lamp until you find the switch. You turn it on.

"Cool!" you think, noticing that the room that will be your castle for the night is well-appointed. The furniture appears to be Henredon, and the room also hosts several beautiful Persian rugs that, given your knowledge of the finer things in life, you recognize as having been constructed Istanbul. You had purchased rugs very similar to these during your recent trip to Turkey. You know that these rugs were not inexpensive.

Your entire experience of the room has been transformed. This room has shifted from a pitch-black cave whose only gift to you was that of hosting your travel-beaten body for the night, to a beautiful well-appointed room that is, for you, a place that is worthy of your presence not only for the time that you will sleep, but also for the time that you wake up in the new day. In fact, for several moments you convince yourself that it will be wonderful to be able to explore this space in greater detail in the morning – after you've concluded several additional hours of sleep – which you still desperately need.

What is the difference between the pre-bathroom experience of the room, the one where you existed in total darkness – and the later experience where you had discovered the light? AWARENESS, of course.

The entrance of awareness in your experience was indeed transformative. Without awareness, the room in which you were resident could have been any flea-bag dump for the evening. With awareness, you discovered the beautiful intricacies of the room – making you appreciate it all the more and regretting the fact that, within the next few hours, you'll be leaving the room to achieve your business objectives, and ultimately go home.

The executive's Gestalt, then, is awakened by awareness: attending to a variety of factors in one's environment that, through even limited attention, can inform the executive to move in one direction or another. Awareness is transformative. Awareness is irreplaceable to the rich and full development of the executive's Gestalt.

The process of awakening the executive Gestalt begins with the senses: the means through which we engage in the world outside of ourselves. These senses connect us with that which is real – and that which can be accessed not only through ourselves and our senses, but also through the selves and the senses of others. Part of the power of the awareness that is available to us is that this same awareness is also available to others – to the degree that they choose to awaken it.

Figure 4: The senses are gateways of awareness.

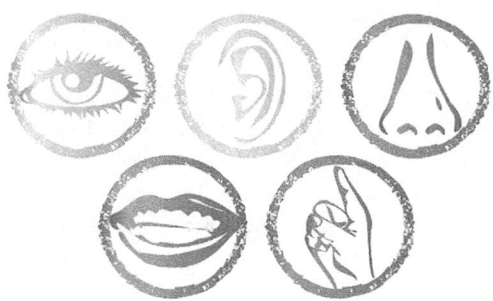

We have available to us five senses that include:
- The eyes – through which we take in such factors as color, size, shape, texture, and location (whether near or far);
- The ears – through which an individual can access auditory information. Sounds: whether loud or soft, high or low are available through the ears. Melodies are also available, through which individuals can be moved, emotionally, stimulated, or calmed;
- The nose – that make olfactory information available to us. Smells such as freshly-baked breads, a perfectly-formed rose, or a field of jasmine, can all be better known to us through our olfactory senses;
- The touch – which allows us to determine texture, size, depth, temperature, and information of this nature, can be accessed through our appendages, or virtually through any place on our bodies where nerves are present;
- The mouth or sense of taste reveals to us things that are bitter, sweet, salty – things that may appeal to us and those things that may not appeal to us.

These senses operate in concert with one another. So when I purchase a large scoop of strawberry ice cream in a waffle cone, I am aware of the coldness of the ice cream, the sweetness of the strawberry flavor, the texture of the strawberry that is embedded in the ice cream, the crunchiness of the waffle cone, and the drip of the ice cream as it melts off of my cone and onto my leg. All of these senses conspire together to create the "strawberry ice cream in waffle cone" experience for us that is a multisensory experience worthy of its own independent description. The sentences here do not give this exciting treat its just desserts.

Activating The Executive's Gestalt

Stepping into the greater fullness of reality that the "Gestalt" offers requires the executive to make many important choices.

First, the executive has to choose to **slow down**. Deepening one's awareness is based on slowing down your traditional routine in such a way that you can see hear, feel, taste, touch, smell things that you may not experience in the past. This slowing down sets your sense up to experience things that were previously unavailable to you. You can now more fully "take in" the unique characteristics of what you're observing.

Figure 5: "Both-and" thinking stimulates the executive's Gestalt.

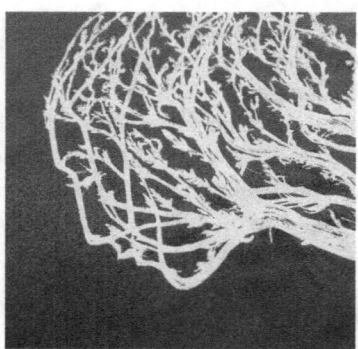

Imagine for a moment that you are driving through a beautiful forest of white birch trees in New Hampshire. You may have been on this road numerous times in the past, but someone was telling you what a beautiful route this was. Upon reflection, you realize that you may have never really paid attention to the trees on the route. Now you do. You might notice countless things that you never attended to before. Despite the fact that these are all white birch trees, you are able to discriminate between them in ways that deepen your appreciation for the beauty of the birch tree and, despite the fact that they are all of the same species, the ways in which these trees distinguish themselves.

Second, the executive must choose to **notice**. Allow your curiosity to simply wander. You may not focus it in any particular direction – just allow your attention to be drawn to whatever it is drawn to. Just let it happen. In the previous example of the birch trees, you might notice the varied heights of the trees, the varied diameters of the trees, or the fact that some of the trees seem to have more bark than others. The goal is not to be wedded to any particular observation – just allow your "noticer" to notice.

Third, you may look deeper – notice **the things that you didn't notice the first time**. No judgements about what you noticed or didn't – just an observation.

Fourth, notice **the patterns or consistency of the things you noticed**. How do the things you noticed fit together? Any familiar themes or patters.

Fifth, notice **the patters or consistency of the things you didn't notice**. While a young executive at Sprint, one of my mentors, whom I'll call "Bob" (since that was his name) asked me, "Ollie, what's it like to be a black leader in this organization?" Thinking on his question for his moment, I responded, "Bob, what's it like to be a white leader in this organization?" Bob's startled non-verbal response spoke volumes. "I never thought about it," came his response. "Therein, my friend, is one of the differences between being black and being white in this organization." In that brief exchange, Bob came to grips with one of the factors that he had never noticed in his own experience of being a white leader in the organization. Bob and I had several additional conversations about that experience we shared – all with him noticing things he had never noticed about being himself in the organization and imagining how my experience of being me in the organization might be different. He was often more insightful than he was willing to give himself credit.

Accelerating the Executive's Gestalt

The greater the executive's ability to accelerate his or her Gestalt, as described here, the greater will be his or her ability to see things previously unseen, to hear things previously unheard, and to engage in areas of his or her life and work in ways that previously did not occur. In other words, the executive's ability to grow, to develop, and to have an even greater impact that he or she has had in the past is very much dependent upon developing the skills that have been described in this chapter.

Figure 6: Holding multiple realities expands the executive's Gestalt.

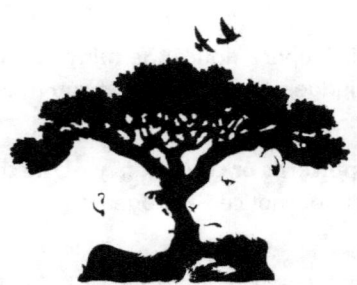

Fundamentally, accelerating the executive's Gestalt is a set of learned and practiced behaviors. As the executive pays attention to those things that he or she did not notice in the past, greater information becomes available. The presence of this additional data makes new choices available to the executive that were not available in the past.

As a result of this expanded number of options that are available to the executive, he or she greatly expands the range of actions that are possible. Rather than doing that which is habitual, familiar, and routine, the executive can now consider other possible alternatives for action.

These expanded options and the ability to make informed decisions about what the executive would choose to do create the foundation for greater information, greater growth, and greater impact.

The executive, and those around him or her, have infinite capacity available to them. As the executive increases his or her ability to see and access the capacity around him or her, and encourages others to do so, individuals and systems grow and continue to grow.

Figure 7: The executive may give no obvious evidence of change, yet expanded awareness may create a "third eye."

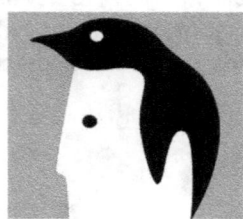

Expanding the Executive's Gestalt

One of the clear benefits of an expanded Gestalt lies in information and perspectives being available that were not previously. As a result, the executive who works with those around them to expand their executive Gestalt opens the possibility for:
1. Greater understanding of the complex realities facing the individual, the team, or the organization;
2. Richer understanding of the range of possibilities for addressing the challenges being faced;
3. Individual, team, and organizational growth that is well beyond an evolutionary pace – as more information is available, greater choices are available, and more collective energy is available for action.

Nevis (1987, p. 69) argues that the consultant's presence creates a learning model, suggesting that expanding the executive Gestalt is not a matter of fireside chats, lengthy seminars, or high-tuition workshops (although there is nothing wrong with these). Nevis's notion is that the intervention of the well-grounded and well-focused individual creates a model (a "presence") worthy of emulation.

Figure 8: Expanding the executive Gestalt raises levels of performance for individuals, teams, and for the entire organization.

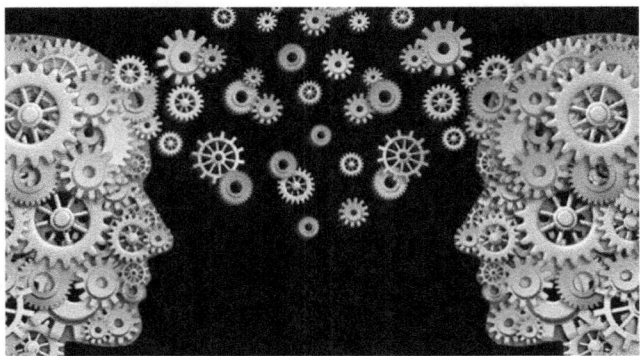

The creation of a revolution in the evolution of the executive's Gestalt may, then, be a function of quiet, focused and centered revolutionaries, rather than leaders with walls, torches, or muskets.

Indeed, the world needs more leaders – at all levels. This chapter argues that the leadership needed is not a caveman, club-on-the-head type of leadership, but leadership borne out of the awareness and intentional action of the informed leader. Armed with her or his fully-formed executive Gestalt, he or she is able to support others in this higher state of informed awareness and action.

References

Anderson, R.J., and William A. Adams (2016). *Mastering leadership*. Hoboken, NJ: John Wiley & Sons.

The Arbinger Institute (2002). *Leadership and self-deception*: Getting out of the box. San Francisco: Berrett-Koehler Publishers, Inc.

Drucker, P.F. (2002). *The effective executive*. New York: Harper Business Essentials.

Gilbert, R. M. (1992). *Extraordinary relationships*: A new way of thinking about human interactions. New York: John Wiley & Sons.

Gilbert, R. M. (2006). *Extraordinary leadership*: Thinking systems, making a difference. Falls Church and Bayse, VA: Leading Systems Press.

Nevis, E. (1987). *Organizational consulting: A Gestalt approach*. New York: Garner Press, Inc.

Patterson, K., Grenny, J., Maxfield, D., McMillan, R., and Switzler, A. (2008). *Influencer*: The power to change anything. New York: McGraw-Hill.

Warner, C. T. (2001). *Bonds that make us free*. Shadow Mountain.

Whitney, D., Trosten-Bloom, A., and Rader, K. (2010). *Appreciative leadership*: focus on what works to drive winning performance and build a thriving organization. New York: McGraw-Hill.

Chapter 10: I'm Better When I Move: Facilitating Movement and Energy in Groups from a Gestalt Perspective

Walt Hopkins

"I'm better when I move" is the story of my lifetime journey as a Gestalt practitioner using movement in groups. It is a story of how I keep learning to spend more time moving – and less time getting lost in my head trying to think things out – and how I keep supporting and teaching participants of groups to do the same. I offer and define seven key principles that have been effective in getting me out of my head sooner: use of energy; sensations – emotions – thoughts; use of self; presence; use of group; noticing; and resistance. I am intentionally writing in first person and present tense.

1. Use of Energy: Red, Blue, Green, Purple

It's midnight. I'm standing alone in the softly-lit Green Room at Eynsham Hall, near Oxford in England. I'm reviewing the row of flipchart easels that I will use with a group tomorrow morning. I've just finished creating these charts in four colours: red, blue, green, and purple. Tomorrow I will explain to the group how each of these colours represents an energy to use in communicating with others.

But now it is time to rehearse. As I have done for decades since I first developed this Gestalt-based approach to movement work, I move through each flipchart in turn and I say aloud what I plan to say in the morning. In addition to rehearsing the words, I am rehearsing the movements that go with each chart. I am moving myself into each movement, just as I will invite the participants to move into each movement in the morning.

Figure 1: Movement and Energy

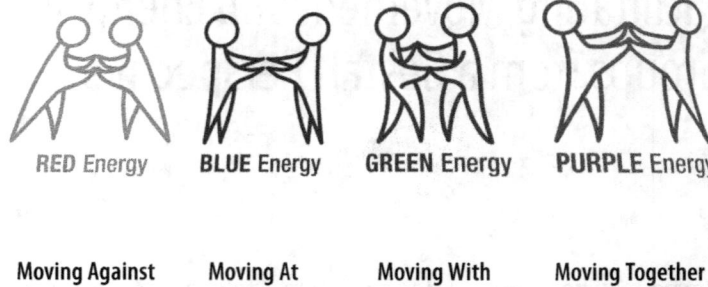

It's morning. I reveal the first chart with its bright red image of two people using RED Energy. I go to the chair where I have stacked shirts in the four different colours, and I pull on the red one. I ask for a volunteer wearing red. I ask the volunteer to put one foot back as a brace and to then put up both hands and push on my hands – just like the image on the chart in Figure 1. Then I ask the whole group to find partners and do the same thing. Some laughter, some hesitation – and now we are moving.

2. Sensations – Emotions – Thoughts

Now I ask people to do the energy exercise again – this time with mouth shut and mind open – and to notice three things. Easily remembered by tennis players, these are the "Three SET Points: **S**ensations, **E**motions, and **T**houghts." What do you notice as **Sensations** in your body such as tension, fatigue, relaxation, calmness, imbalance, balance? What do you notice as **Emotions** connected to those Sensations such as confusion, happiness, sadness, anxiety, excitement, relief? What do you notice as **Thoughts** about what is going on such as strange, funny, puzzling, challenging, boring, stimulating? (Hopkins 2012, p. 113)

I ask for one-word descriptions of the Sensations, Emotions, and Thoughts that people notice. I write them – in red – on a flipchart and then I use the wide range of reactions to point out Three SET Points of learnings from the experience:
1. You experience these Sensations, Emotions, and Thoughts even though you are not talking during the exercise.
2. Different people have different – even opposite – Sensations,

Emotions, and Thoughts while using the same energy.
3. You may have positive experiences with an energy that other people have negative experiences with energy. So while you may feel comfortable using that energy, the other person may feel uncomfortable. And vice versa. (Hopkins 2012, p. 114)

After we gather the SET words, I introduce the Energy: This is **RED Energy** or what I also call Moving Against Energy. The first movement of RED Energy is **Demanding**, as in "I want...."

Now the volunteer and I demonstrate the other half of RED Energy. We begin with our hands pushing against each other as before. Then I decrease the pressure with one hand and increase it with the other. Our arms go back and forth. After the whole group does this, I again ask for Three SET Points. The second movement of RED Energy is **Exchanging**, as in "If you...then I..." Putting the two movements of RED Energy together creates a result: Demanding + Exchanging = Deal (Table A).

ENERGY: COLOR, DIRECTION, MOVEMENTS, RESULTS				
Color	Energy Direction	Movement 1: Ways to 'Say' What I Want	Movement 2: Ways to 'Get' What I Want	Four Results
Red	Moving Against	Demanding	Exchanging	Deal
Blue	Moving At	Proposing	Reasoning	Solution
Green	Moving With	Sharing	Listening	Understanding
Purple	Moving Together	Envisioning	Connecting	Cooperation

Table A: Four Energies

Now I reach for the blue shirt and go through the same process for BLUE, then GREEN, and then PURPLE. Each time, we experience the two Movements of each Energy that equal a Result. BLUE Energy: Proposing + Reasoning = Solution. GREEN Energy: Sharing + Listening = Understanding. PURPLE Energy: Envisioning + Connecting = Cooperation.

I say to the group, "If I had just given a lecture on the energies – instead of getting you up and moving first – and then asking for your reactions, I'd be getting a lot of resistance. The beauty of working with body movement in a group is that you and the other participants are doing your own research in the here and now with your most trusted source: yourself."

That is why I begin with movement rather than talking about it. If someone wants proof that these energies work, then Perls, Hefferline, and Goodman offer the perfect response: "…we present nothing that you cannot *verify for yourself in terms of your own behaviour.*" (1951, p. 7). I also refer to *Alice's Adventures in Wonderland* (Carroll 1865): "The best way to explain it is to do it."

When I finish introducing a group to the Energy Model, I encourage people to "keep it in mind" and then – in my ongoing attempt to add a new phrase to the language – I also encourage people to "keep it in body" as a way of remembering the experience of each energy.

Use of Self: My Own Journey Into Using Movement In Groups

It's evening – a long time ago in a country far, far away. I am in my late twenties. It's the first year of my first training programme at the Gestalt Institute of Cleveland (GIC). I am talking in the group – but not getting anywhere. I make a note about our trainer, Janet Leon who is trying to get me to move. I'm beginning the long journey to discovering that moving helps.

But first I invest a lot of energy in resisting the whole idea of moving. And I keep getting nowhere. Eventually, some weeks later in the group, I risk moving briefly and Janet sighs in relief. I've begun to move.

Use of self means to me that I make use *now* of how I have resisted in the *past* – as part of my own learning. Now I can honour resistance in groups as members begin learning the same things.

It's another evening a year later. In another training group at GIC, Gestalt therapist Miriam (Mim) Polster is working with our group on dreams. I offer a recent dream: I am swimming in the lake and approaching a pier. I am worn out and need help to get out of the water. United States President Nixon is on the pier and refuses to help me out.

I talk about how I see a connection between this dream and the foundation that just rejected my grant application. Mim moves me away from talking *about* it and into movement. She offers me an experiment – an experience in which we co-create what happens. Mim gradually scales up the experiment, checking with me as we go. Mim reminds us of the "safe emergency" in which the person doing the work pays attention to both ends of that continuum with two questions: Am I getting enough support to feel **safe** in doing this experiment? Am I feeling enough **risk** in doing this that I think I might learn something? (Polster and Polster 1973, pp. 234-235)

Mim encourages the rest of the group to get involved. Some members of the group provide chairs and cushions as needed. One group member Joan volunteers to take the role of Nixon on the pier, saying that she wants to learn how it feels to be like Nixon.

Mim then suggests that I swim. Forty-five years later, I still feel the soft roughness of the carpet as I do a crawl stroke across the floor to the pier and see Nixon towering over me (Joan is standing on a chair). Nixon tells me I cannot come out of the water. I keep holding on and hoping. Joan, as Nixon, screams down at me that by asking her permission, I give her power and she will never give me anything. I will have to get it myself. Eventually, I ignore Nixon and stop asking for help. I pull myself up on my own and I walk past Nixon into my own future. (Hopkins 1974, p. 90)

I'm Better When I Move

Several years before I began learning about Gestalt, I saw a movie with a memorable scene about moving: *Butch Cassidy and the Sundance Kid*. In a long conversation with my lifetime friend Johnny King – after we watched the film again recently – I realised that my favourite scene in the film matches my own experience.

While looking at Sundance's gun, a man tosses his tobacco pouch 30 yards away, and challenges Sundance to hit it. Sundance tries to put the gun back in his holster, but the man insists that he just point it. Sundance aims – and misses. Then he says to the man, "Can I move?"

"Move? What the hell you mean, move?"

Sundance draws, hits the pouch on the ground – and again in the air. In the best tradition of a laconic cowboy, he then says, "I'm better when I move."

"I'm better when I move" is my lifetime learning as a Gestalt practitioner. I can still get lost in my head, lost in my words, lost in hanging on too long, lost in trying to figure it all out. The difference now is that I can get out of my head sooner – sometimes just by taking a walk. I'm better when I move.

Presence

When I am working in groups – and especially when I am doing movement and energy work with groups – I need to establish my **Presence** and share my **Use of Self**. As Gestalt consultants Mary Ann Rainey and Jonno Hanafin explain, "Presence represents the translation of personal appearance, manner, values, knowledge, reputation, and other characteristics into interest and impact…. Presence is use of self with intent." (Rainey Tolbert and Hanafin, 2006, p.72)

Establishing **Presence** begins as I arrive in a group. I learned this from Sonia Nevis, my mentor at the Gestalt Institute of Cleveland (variably GIC and the Institute). When I co-trained my first weekend workshop at GIC with Sonia, I was very nervous. I put on my favourite purple shirt to feel a bit better. When I walked into the Institute, Sonia was coming out of her office – wearing a gorgeous long purple dress. I commented delightedly on our synchronicity. She calmly responded, "Of course. Purple is for power and passion. That is what we are here for."

When I created my energy model for influencing, I chose a colour for each energy. PURPLE Energy is the energy of power and passion. In 2012, when I published my book about influencing, Sonia wrote to say: "Such a good book – you are probably as proud of it as I am proud of you." (Nevis, S., 2012, *Personal correspondence*) The cover of the book is **purple**.

When I pull on the purple shirt while demonstrating PURPLE Energy, I remember Sonia and me wearing purple. Both then and now, I am establishing Presence through Rainey and Hanafin's "use of self with intent." (Rainey Tolbert and Hanafin, 2006, p.72)

Use of Group

As I make Use of Self, I also make **Use of Group**. When someone in the group says, "I've been sitting too long; I need to move," I could just watch them stand by the window or I could just begin thinking of some group movement I could offer.

Instead, I make use of Use of Group by wondering aloud if someone in the group has a way we can all move. Recently, this Use of Group has led to several different forms of group movement, each led by a member of the group, ranging from lively dancing to a slowly flowing tai chi routine. The challenge is to let the group do the work. If they are doing it, then I can just stay out of the way.

Other times, we do Use of Self and Use of Group together – as group and trainer. You can imagine that you are in a group, telling the group that you feel unsupported in your life. The others in the group start talking with you about how they support you. This is all words. Time to move.

As we begin developing an experiment, I remind us all (including myself) that we are here to Care for you in your experiment and to Dare you to find the right level of Safe Risk – my shorter version of what the Polsters call the Safe Emergency. (Polster and Polster 1973, pp. 234-235)

As much as we may want to Care or Dare, you are the final arbiter of your own Safe Risk. You are already lying on the floor because at least the floor is supporting you. Someone suggests that we physically show how we support you – by lifting you from the floor. As we are scaling up the experiment, I review the Safe Risk again with you AND with the rest of the group. I scale the Risk down by suggesting we only lift you four inches off the floor.

Now I make very sure that you are supported all the way around, with the strongest people above your waist and at your head. Some people check their own level of Safe Risk and shift places. I am assessing your weight before deciding that the risk for us and for you is safe enough. In any case, I am at or near your head so that I can keep both an eye and a hand on you.

We rehearse the lift and then we do it. We hold you in the air – just a few inches above the floor – and then return you safely to earth. After the shining eyes and before the conversation, I use two of my more frequent words in a T (training) Group: "Sloooow down." After intense work, we need to pause and breathe. I suggest that you use your journals to reflect on what you have learned. For these intense experiences, I offer **Seven Quick Bits** as ways for journaling concisely about what's most important at the moment. (Hopkins 2017, p.13)

Much Ado About Noticing

I often begin a group with a flipchart that says *Much Ado About Nothing* and then I share my favourite learning about this play. Shakespeare loved puns and he uses one in this title. In the English of his day, the word "nothing" was pronounced more like "noting" and this play is full of characters leaning around a corner to notice what other people are doing. I frame the week ahead as much ado about **noticing**. I'm going to be noticing, and I'm encouraging you to notice too.

During the past fifty years, I have participated in hundreds of groups, and facilitated hundreds more. Some are T Groups, some are management teams, and some are volunteer groups. In all these groups, I use at least some of my Gestalt training at least some of the time. With two of the groups recently, I made a small intervention that changed how those groups have worked ever since. In both cases, I **noticed** that the meeting room was set up with a head table for the leaders facing rows of chairs for everyone else. I simply suggested that we move the chairs into a circle. One of the goals in Gestalt work is enabling people to move into contact. That is easier, as well as much more likely, when each of us can **see** and **be seen**.

Just as I finished writing the previous paragraph, a colleague from one of those groups, Sheila, stopped in for a chat. I mentioned that I had been writing about that small intervention. Sheila reacted instantly, "That was **not** a small intervention! It transformed the group four years ago and has kept us going since then."

I do a lot of noticing without intervening. As American baseball catcher and manager Yogi Berra said to his baseball players, "You can observe a lot by watching." (Berra 1998, p. 95)

Moving With Resistance

Resistance happens often in groups. Here is another opportunity for Use of Self. I know about resistance from years of doing it so thoroughly during my Gestalt training. I haven't stopped resisting, but I do recognise it a lot faster. So when someone starts resisting, I am ready. I could present a lecture on my seven learnings about resistance. Or we could move.

Here's how it might begin: Imagine you are in a group and sound frustrated, "I don't know what to do. That person just keeps resisting me." Other people in the room begin offering you advice. I'm tempted to offer my own advice, so I go into my head. My head is a nice place to be – I spend a lot of time there. However, as the neuroscientist Antonio Damasio points out, it is your body that actually provides the ongoing stream of data that enables your physical brain to create what we like to call the mind: "Moment by moment, the brain has available a dynamic representation of an entity with a limited range of possible states – the body." (Damasio 2000, p. 142) Your body gives you a lot of information – if you pay attention.

So once again, I move out of my head – and I ask you to stand up with me. I hold up my hand with the palm facing toward you. You take the hint and do the same. I put my hand against yours. You accept that. I put on some pressure. You do the same. Then I ask the rest of the group to stand with a partner and do what we have just done – and then do it again with the opposite person putting pressure on first. I ask what you noticed. You all noticed that you pushed back.

Now that you have the feel of resistance, I share my Seven Learnings about Resistance from my many years of resisting, as well as being resisted. (Hopkins 2012, pp. 15-22)

1. Resistance is **Normal**.
   You resist instinctively. So does everyone else. It's normal. Even if you gave a bit of ground, at some point you stopped and pushed back. It's normal.
2. Resistance is an **Alert**
   When you sense resistance from someone else or within yourself, this is an alert to pay special attention. Notice that **both** of you are resisting.
3. Resistance is an **Iceberg**.
   Even small surface hints of resistance (from others or within you) may be clues to much deeper resistance below. Explore with care – paying attention to cultural differences.
4. Resistance is **Contact**.
   Again we begin with an exercise. I put pressure on your hand and ask you to remove your hand suddenly. Even though I brace myself, I may still stagger at first.
   If someone walks away from you, you can do nothing. But if someone resists you, you are in contact and you can continue to work.
5. Resistance is an **Opportunity**.
   If you are resisting something, you have energy and you can learn from what you are resisting. If I'm resisting you, then you can listen to me and find out more about my resistance. If I don't have to defend myself against your attack, I can change much more easily.
6. **Pay Attention** to the resistance.
   When you sense resistance in yourself or others, pay careful attention to what you are thinking and feeling. You might discover that the resistance is more complicated than you

149

thought. Ed Nevis and his colleagues offer this possibility with their comment on multiple realities: "Another reason for a more respectful reaction to realities other than one's own is that resistance is not an all-or-nothing but rather is best seen as ambivalence." (Nevis, Lancourt, Vassalo 1996, p. 60.)

7. **Move With** the resistance.

We begin with the original exercise of palm against palm. Then I let you push me backward. I step backward a few steps, moving with your energy as you continue to push me. I notice that although we are going in **your** direction, we are at least **moving**. That opens up possibilities. As we keep moving I begin drifting to the left and gradually we change direction. If I keep doing that, we can end up moving in my direction after all. Or perhaps we move in a direction that neither of us had chosen originally.

If you stop moving against me, I can still move myself around to stand beside you. From that position I am more able to see things from your perspective. That might encourage me to change my approach. Or maybe we both will. (Hopkins 2012, pp. 15-22)

After we have been through the seven learnings, I ask you to stand with the person who has been resisting you. You do the first step with each other. I point out that both of you are now resisting and both of you now have the opportunity to move with the other, instead of resisting each other.

We are approaching the end of this version of my learnings about using movement and energy in groups. Just as I would in a group, I have shared the four **Energies** of RED, BLUE, GREEN, and PURPLE, as well as the **Three SET Points**. I have shared stories of **Use of Self** – with intent – to establish **Presence**. I have shared stories about involving participants in **Use of Group** by encouraging Much Ado about **Noticing**. And finally, we have moved through the seven learnings about **Resistance**.

In a group, this gradual process of experiencing all these ways of using movement and energy, makes it possible for us to do experiments later in the week that build on all those movement experiences. Let's imagine how it might happen.

You are talking about how you are trying to reach a goal, but other people are blocking your way. Some members of the group are giving you advice. I ask if you are willing to do an experiment. You say yes.

I review Safe Risk with you and review Care and Dare with everyone. I ask if you play any sports and you say football. We scale up an experiment with a cushion for a ball and two chairs to define the goal. I challenge you to make your goal. My long-forgotten brief time as a goalie re-emerges, and I block several attempts. By this time, the group is cheering you on and you are becoming more determined to score – while I am getting better at blocking. When you finally do score the goal, you are totally energised and ready to move toward your real goal. I encourage you to note how are feeling now so you can keep it in body and return to that energised feeling each time you need to encourage yourself to move on your goal.

The group bursts into spontaneous dancing in celebration of your success – and then more dancing in celebration of our learnings as a flowing, growing group.

Like Sundance, we are all better when we move.

References

Berra, Y. (1998). *The Yogi Book: I Really Didn't Say Everything I Said*. New York: Workman, p. 95.

Butch Cassidy and the Sundance Kid 1969, film. Twentieth Century Fox.

Carroll, L. (1865). *Alice's Adventures in Wonderland*. 1961 reprint London: Folio Society, London.

Damasio, A. (2000). *The Feeling of What Happens: Body, Emotion, and the Making of Consciousness*. London: Vintage, p. 142

Hopkins, W. (1974). Book 25: *The Making of a Learning Consultant, Project Demonstrating Excellence Worthy of a Ph.D.*, Yellow Springs, OH: Union Graduate School, p.90.

Hopkins, W. (2012). *Influencing for Results in Organisations*. Faringdon, Oxfordshire: Libri.

Hopkins, W. (2014). *Influencing for Results in Organisations: 7 videos on how to Influence for Results*, http://www.walthopkins.com/en/influencing-tools/videos/

Hopkins, W. (2017). *Journaling Passport*, Faringdon, Oxfordshire: Libri, p. 13.

Nevis, E., Lancourt, J., & Vassalo, H.G. (1996). *Intentional Revolutions: A Seven-Point Strategy for Transforming Organizations*. San Francisco, CA: Jossey-Bass, p. 60.

Nevis, S. (2012). *Handwritten personal correspondence*.

Perls, F., Hefferline, R.F., & Goodman, P. (1951). *Gestalt Therapy: Excitement and Growth in the Human Personality*. New York: Delta, p.7.

Polster, E. & Polster, M. (1973). *Gestalt Therapy Integrated: Contours of Theory & Practice*. New York: Brunner/Mazel, pp. 234-235.

Rainey Tolbert, M.A. & Hanafin, J. (2006). "Use of self in OD consulting: What matters is presence." In B. B. Jones & M. Brazzel (Eds.), *The NTL handbook of organization development and change: Principles, practices, and perspectives*. San Francisco, CA: Pfeiffer.

Chapter 11: The Cape Cod Model in Organizational Settings

Joseph Melnick

Introduction

This chapter presents a brief introduction to the Cape Cod Model of Change as it is practiced in organizational settings. It is holistic and incorporates a view of the self; our biological wiring; perceptual and organizational apparatus. Our personalities, how we behave in intimate and task oriented systems are all connected. The Model has its roots in the Center for Intimacy, a former division of the Gestalt Institute of Cleveland (GIC). The Center focused on teaching practitioners to work with small systems such as couples and families. As its reputation grew, the program began to attract executives, coaches, and organizational consultants who found that its principles had relevance for organizations.

We eventually separated from GIC, and created our own institute, the Gestalt International Study Center (GISC) in Cape Cod, Massachusetts, USA, where we continued to develop the Model (Melnick & Nevis, S., 2018).*

The Cape Cod Model is used with therapists, consultants, coaches, leaders, and organizations, and is taught throughout the world in a variety of programs. It is more than a model for working with small systems. It is a philosophy, grounded in Gestalt theory that supports the building of robust relationships and living a good life. Below is a summary of some of its underpinnings (Melnick & Nevis, S., 2018).

- Awareness offers the opportunity to change. When something becomes a habit, we are no longer aware of what we are doing. For example, most of us are not aware of how we brush our

---

* The long term faculty consisted of Stephanie Backman, MSW; Joseph Melnick, Ph.D, Sonia Nevis, Ph.D., and Joseph Zinker, Ph.D. They were joined by Edwin Nevis, Ph.D., whom many consider to be the founder of Gestalt Organizational Development.

teeth, drive our car, eat our food or talk to each other. When we become aware, we notice. Only when we notice do we have a choice between making a change or doing things as we always have.
- Sometimes awareness can lead to depression and sadness, as when we become aware of pain or we become aware of wants that cannot be fulfilled.
- Some of us pay attention to thoughts first and others first to emotions. To live well in the world, we have to be able to attend to both. Competency involves an ability to be in touch with both thoughts and emotions and being able to think and feel before acting.
- We all carry the past forever within us. The future – including our hopes, wishes, plans, fantasies, and daydreams – also exists, yet we cannot live in the past or the future as much as we would sometimes like. The *now* is all we really have.
- The future is always unknown. We do not know what the next second, day, or year will bring.
- Every experience is composed of many ingredients that shift as a function of the moment and of the situation. It is the situation that is the primary organizer of experience, but most of the time it does not feel that way.
- Whenever two or more people are interacting – working together or talking to each other – whatever happens has been crafted by all involved. As simple as it sounds, it is a radical departure from how most of us understand our process.
- Every habit – whether good or bad – was used initially to solve a problem. Most of our habits continue to be useful. Some, however, are no longer productive, but we continue to use them anyway. This is true for both individuals and organizations.
- Resisting can be useful or useless. Competency involves knowing when to say yes and when to say no; when to act and when to wait; when to try new things; and when to stick with the old.
- Few of us has ever awoken saying, "I am going to mess up my day". Most of us are doing the best we can, even when things don't work out as we had expected or hoped.
- Even the best of us messes up often. To turn against ourselves after we err is rarely useful. Mistakes are ordinary.
- Nobody owns the truth. We all see things differently. Competent behavior involves a willingness to talk and listen to

others who are different or who have different points of view.
- Power is neither good nor bad, nor does it exist solely within individuals, but rather *between* people, groups, organizations, and even nations.
- Most of our relationships contain some form of hierarchy whether implicit or explicit. Hierarchy needs to be acknowledged and respected and the rules for clear communication understood by all. The health of a hierarchical system such as an organization depends on the relational competence of those in the hierarchy.
- We are always having impact, both good and bad, depending on how we present ourselves to others. We call our self-presentation *presence* (Melnick, J. & Nevis, E., 2012).
- Maturity, in part, involves creating lives that are filled with possibilities. We are able to move towards things that have potential, to feel regret when things don't turn out as expected, and to move on, having learned from the experience.
- Growth and development come from our movement toward what is different from the way we are.[*]

Important Conceptual Constructs

Optimism

Lately, there has been a tremendous emphasis on optimism in organizational consultation, along with a focus on the positive – on what people are doing well, as opposed to their failures. Many contemporary organizational approaches such as Appreciative Inquiry (Cooperrider, Sorensen, Whitney, & Yaeger, 2000) also embrace this perspective. The benefits of a focus on the positive are supported by much research that indicates that people who are optimistic live longer, are healthier both physically and psychologically, and are more successful and resilient (Melnick & Nevis, S., 2016).

Now, of course, there is also an important place for pessimism in our lives. By pessimism I mean a focus on potential threats and concern for potential danger. Most of us want this perspective in our lawyers and surgeons. We also want it in ourselves when walking down a dark street

---

[*] A more formal description of our core concepts can be found in Melnick and Nevis, S. (2018) Appendix A.

at midnight in a high crime district, or when considering a potential risky stock investment. It is a closed, tense, suspicious and focused stance, one in which we are "looking for trouble." The advantage of being able to appropriately embrace this attitude is that you won't be surprised by actual danger. The disadvantage, when overused, is that you might not notice new opportunities and potential.

We should point out that by optimism we are not talking of the naive type, found in immature people who believe that young love will naturally last forever without hard work, or who expect to win the lottery. In organizational work, it is important to realistically look for threats, but if this looking is overdone, it will lead to unnecessary anxiety, and diminish the potential for joy and creativity.

Whether working with small systems or large organizations our model focuses on what is working well. An optimistic stance incorporates a belief that no matter what happens in the next moment, we will have the resources and the resilience to deal with it. This stance allows us to move beyond the habitual and to try new things.

Cycle of Experience

The founders of the Gestalt Institute of Cleveland created a visual template for describing the flow of energy and named it the Cycle of Experience (COE). Originally taken from the work of Perls and Goodman (Perls, Hefferline & Goodman, 1951) it summarized the process by which people, either individually or collectively, become aware of what is going on at a given movement. It describes how they mobilize energy to act, engage, make meaning, and assimilate new experiences (Nevis, E., 1987). Originally described as a cycle, it is in fact more a sine wave that can be artificially divided into *sensation, awareness, mobilization, action, meaning making and withdrawal*, with *contact* occurring at all stages (Melnick & Nevis, S. 2018). In working with more than one person, it is important that individual cycles be synchronized before moving to action.

Let me give you two quick examples. The first involves a group of trial attorneys who, when viewed through the COE, favored mobilization and action over sensation and awareness. In their training as lawyers, they were taught to privilege advocacy over inquiry. Never *ask a question to which you don't know the answer*.

They were frustrated with their corporate meetings and unable to reach decisions that *stuck*. Once they became aware that their cultural strength as trial lawyers was problematic in their meetings, they adopted a slogan, *Connection before action*. They began starting their meetings with check-ins in which all the attorneys said a few words about their personal and professional lives and the practice as a whole before addressing the agenda. It has been more than ten years since they adopted this way of starting and it has transformed not only their meetings but how they function as a group.

A second example concerns a physician organization that complained that their meetings dissolved into chaos. They did not have good endings in their meetings partially due to the fact that the physicians were often overbooked with overlapping meetings. As a result, there was rarely time for closure and meaning making as the physicians would begin to inch towards the door prior to the actual end of the meetings. One outcome of this pattern was that a significant portion of each meeting was spent helping the "early leavers" catch up to what was agreed upon previously. In order to address this problem they agreed upon the following "rules." First, all cell phones and pagers needed to be turned off, and coverage needed to be found. Second, everyone needed to stay until the completion of the meeting. And third, the meaning making portion of the meeting, including agreements and next steps, would begin two-thirds into the meeting to allow time for a more complete and aesthetic ending.

Change

As dictated by the Paradoxical Theory of Change (Beisser, 1970), awareness of what we are doing (at the individual, dyadic, work group, or organizational level) leads to choice and the potential for change. Change rarely occurs by elimination, but instead involves the addition of new habits and behaviors. Rather than teaching our clients to get rid of bothersome patterns, we first teach them to become interested in what they are doing. Once they learn that every pattern, no matter how "good" or "bad" was originally created to solve a problem and has a nugget of competence in it, they can then look at the price they pay for its overuse.

Resistance

We understand that as change agents, when we enter an organization, we often elicit *resistance;* a counter-force – dedicated to keeping things the same, no matter how bad they are. By resistance, we simply mean that others have different thoughts, values, and life experiences than we do. We understand that there is always a kernel of truth in every resistance, and successfully dealing with it is essential. In fact, if we do not experience resistance, it may go underground, making it more difficult to address.

As Gestalt practitioners we move *towards* the resistance and resister. We join them as we view the resistance as a way to begin to build trust and connection. So, for example, in the lawyer organization mentioned previously, I was confronted by a young associate who detailed how I was "wrong." I welcomed his comments telling him that "It probably was not the first time I was wrong that day." and asked him if he would let me know anytime he questioned something I was saying. He seemed surprised at my response, but quickly agreed. Not only had we begun to establish a trusting relationship, but so had the rest of the group who had been watching carefully as to how I would handle his criticism.

Trust

Trust is necessary for most learning, for when we trust others we can relax and be open to influence. Most consultants generate preliminary trust via their degrees, dress, and resumes. However, a more enduring trust must be earned, for only naive individuals trust quickly. In fact, if trust occurs too quickly, it is a potential sign of trouble up ahead. And, of course, trust is two way, for if we do not trust the individuals, teams and organizations that we work with, we too can't be open to connecting and teaching.

In the Cape Cod Model we build trust in a number of ways. For example, we respond to questions not only in terms of content but as opportunities to create connection. After giving a response, we might add "Did that make sense?" or "Did my answer surprise you?" We notice not only the content, but also body language. We might say "You said you were satisfied, but I thought I picked up some hesitation in your voice. If I did not answer your question, let's try again. "And if, after trying we still cannot answer the question, we acknowledge that fact. Then, if appropriate, we promise to get back to them. When others in the work group see our response, it encourages them to express their curiosity. This approach to question/answer dynamics counteracts the experience of many in school or work settings when the questioner is given just a one-word answer or made to feel ashamed for asking. We understand that completion builds trust, whereas incompletion and disconnection diminishes it.

We don't play favorites, and we don't demonize individuals. We respect all, including those at the top of the hierarchy, for a well-functioning hierarchy is important for the life of the organization (Melnick & Nevis, S., 2018). We minimize "surprise." When we are surprised, we become involuntarily vulnerable, making it difficult to organize a well thought out response, thus losing our ability to respond in an integrated way. Instead, we tell clients how we are going to intervene and the rationale behind our intervention. Then we spend time seeing if it makes sense. And if it does not (resistance?), we deal with the objections in a respectful and joining way. Not only is trust two way, it also waxes and wanes. This is normal and ordinary, and when trust diminishes, we are committed to devoting the time and energy to improve it.

Presence

Our first task is to present ourselves in such a way that interest and trust are generated. Presence is different than charisma, for we all have presence. One might say it is the sum of who we are, our ability to be *present* in the here and now and engage others. When we are present, we are able to creatively respond to a new situation. Presence includes an ability to be flexible in terms of what parts of ourselves we use in responding to situations, often incorporating an ability to be brief and bold and to be friendly with all parts of ourselves.

Mary, a diminutive woman with a small voice, was worried about establishing her presence as she was about to begin consulting to an all-male leadership team, known for their aggressiveness. She consulted her supervisor, asking if he would join her. He declined, saying that if he were in the room, she would always appear the junior consultant. Instead, he suggested that she arrive a few minutes late for their first meeting, select the most aggressive executive, walk up to him, look him in the eye and say, "Excuse me. I believe you are sitting in my chair." She did, he moved, and she quickly established herself.

In our teaching we sometimes break presence into a set of skills. We ask our students to fill out the questionnaire below and give each other feedback in order to analyze which of their skills are well developed and which are less developed.

Table 1

SKILLS THAT ENHANCE PRESENCE	
Please circle the number that reflects your competency.	
Ability to be open and receptive 1 2 3 4 5 Well-Developed Less-Developed	**Ability to separate what you observe from what you think it means** 1 2 3 4 5 Well-Developed Less-Developed
Ability to gauge and embody the appropriate amount of space for the task at hand (language, body language, tone, volume, etc.) 1 2 3 4 5 Well-Developed Less-Developed	**Ability to put things succinctly, clearly, and directly** 1 2 3 4 5 Well-Developed Less-Developed
Ability to stay in the here and now 1 2 3 4 5 Well-Developed Less-Developed	**Ability to embody respect, interest, and curiosity in yourself and the other(s)** 1 2 3 4 5 Well-Developed Less-Developed
Ability to notice and be curious about physical behaviors in yourself and the other(s) 1 2 3 4 5 Well-Developed Less-Developed	**Ability to use and respond to humor** 1 2 3 4 5 Well-Developed Less-Developed
Ability to tune in to your emotions and those of the other(s) 1 2 3 4 5 Well-Developed Less-Developed	**Ability to be bold** 1 2 3 4 5 Well-Developed Less-Developed **Ability to be flexible** 1 2 3 4 5 Well-Developed Less-Developed

Copyright© 2016 Gestalt International Study Center.
All Rights Reserved.

Strategy/Intimacy

Organizations have goals and are designed to produce products and outcomes (strategy). In order to do so, they must create relationships and develop patterns of relating (intimacy). Strategy and intimacy are interwoven in all organizations. Too much of one occurs at the expense of the other and diminishes the organizations or client's capacity to move forward. A good example can be found in the award winning movie, *The King's Speech*, in which an eccentric speech therapist helps the King address his stutter. Although the goal is clear – to help the King diminish or eliminate his stuttering, the path to it is littered with periods of diminished trust and reconciliation, movements between strategic and intimate relating, that are dealt with successfully so that the King can learn and the therapist teach (Melnick & Nevis, S., 2018).

Teaching the Model

We teach the Cape Cod Model as a scaffolding process, a step by step progression that mirrors the Cycle of Experience. Each module is designed to teach specific skills that are incorporated one at a time. Our programs are practice heavy, and participants learn much like a beginning musician learns scales. In time they develop their own style, and their work looks more like jazz; improvisational and responsive to ever changing contexts.

Small Talk

We first engage in "small talk" to allow all to relax in order to begin to create trust and connection, setting the stage for learning. It is essentially a warm up period, much like what sports teams do when they stretch and begin throwing the ball, or when members of an orchestra begin by playing their instruments, first alone and then with others prior to starting the concert.

Instruct the System

In our fast paced world there is often a call for quick solutions and quick interventions. Despite this pressure we spend time explaining our stance. We tell clients how we are going to work with them before we begin, so that they do not have to guess. If they are wondering what is going to happen next, they will not be open to the present moment. We tell them that we are going to sit back and observe them, noticing how they interact and what they are doing well and, at some point, tell them what we heard and saw (Nevis, E., Melnick, & Nevis, S., 2018). Many organizations are not aware of their breath of competencies and may have to be convinced of the value of this focus. It is here that objections and challenges appear. Unlike many models we welcome this "resistance,' viewing it as an opportunity to build trust and connection.

Observe the System

We sit back and look for patterns of connection, appreciating that these are competencies. This form of "seeing" involves an open, relaxed stance; seeing rather than looking, being receptive rather than staring. It incorporates an ability to focus on the interactions of the work team rather than on individuals, and on the *process* rather than the content being discussed. It involves a relaxed stance of waiting until a pattern of interaction emerges. Since most of us (including our clients) are trained to look at deficiencies and what is going wrong, observing competency is a surprisingly difficult skill to learn.

Intervene

By *intervention* we mean a stronger, more potent statement than an ordinary exchange, one that is designed to draw attention to a specific behavioral pattern. The intervention is not about flattery or positive judgments. We do not say "You are a wonderful team" or "You are doing a great job". We point to specific identifiable behaviors, such as "You have been meeting for an hour, everyone has been verbally involved with each of you sitting on the edge of your seat during this entire time." It is often here where we also experience resistance.

Our first interventions are to heighten the awareness of the group's competence so as to free up energy, interest and curiosity. Once we become aware of a pattern or habit, new possibilities emerge, allowing us to do something different. We often use a term "well developed" to categorize these competencies.

Sit Back, Observe Patterns, and Intervene

Once the first intervention has had impact we sit back to see what happens next knowing that every competency (well developed) has its cost. For example, you might notice that the group that has "high energy" – "as you work, all are sitting on the edge of your seats, leaning forward, and speaking quickly and passionately. However, you seldom sit back, take slow breaths and relax". Or, "You are good at agreeing and supporting each other, but we also notice that you seldom disagree." Or, "All of you have the courage to speak your truth regarding a whole range of issues, yet you rarely ask questions of each other."

Create an Experiment, a "Try This"

Experiments are vehicles co-created with clients to heighten awareness and practice a new skill or pattern. The use of experiments draws on a fundamental principle of the Gestalt approach. It is a belief in *embodiment*; i.e., for learning to have long term impact, it must be absorbed – not just cognitively, but also emotionally and physically in our bodies.

End Well

We generally end all sessions with clients by asking them to articulate what they got out of the session and to create next doable steps. This is the meaning making, closure part of the COE (Melnick & Roos, 2007).

Case Study

I recently worked with a leadership team of a large state agency. They had been dealing with large program cuts initiated by a new governor who questioned the department's mission. As they began meeting to deal with the upcoming budget cuts, the group was dealing with high burn out. This included concern for the leader, a highly empathic and relational man who cared deeply for all of them. In addition, two of the members who had been about to retire had decided to stay on after finding out that upon retirement their positions would be eliminated. They could not bear deserting their colleagues.

They were stuck. They couldn't move forward and make some of the hard decisions that were demanded of them. After a series of individual meetings to assess the situation and to establish initial trust and connection, we began meeting to address and deal with the budget cuts.

As I observed them interacting, I noticed many positives. They shared a commitment to the agency's mission, the connection between team members, the active involvement of the leader in all decisions, and the members' respect and concern for the leader. In fact, the leader was usually center stage. Everything seemed to go through them.

Looking back, probably the most valuable intervention was an experiment in which I invited the leader to sit back and join me observing his team. I had the team function without his verbal participation. We became a temporary leadership team, in which, with my support, he would periodically intervene and tell the group what they were doing well. Over time, with the leader sitting back, the group became more relaxed and began to address each other and the issues in creative ways. They developed a plan to deal with the budget cuts. Two members of the team were able to retire and others turned to external coaches for support.

Conclusion

The Cape Cod Model is a Gestalt based approach to organizational intervention. It is a holistic approach incorporating the belief that we move towards symmetry, toward *good form*. Grounded in the Cycle of Experience, it views organizations as essentially a series of patterns and connections. By developing a series of skills, such as how to create trust, intervene, and deal with resistance, the consultant is able to help clients notice their patterns, appreciating the good and bad of them. An optimistic stance, supports them in keeping, diminishing, and adding on to patterns to increase the systems' effectiveness, both relationally and strategically. The model is designed to create situations in which everyone is open to giving and receiving feedback, and to influencing and being influenced. The Cape Cod Model focuses on recognizing competence, thus creating developmental opportunities.

References

Beisser, A. (1970). 'The Paradoxical Theory of Change' in J. Fagan and I. Shepherd, (eds.) *Gestalt Therapy Now: Theory, techniques, and applications* (pp. 77-80). Palo Alto. CA: Science and Behavioral Books.

Cooperrider, D. Sorensen, P. Whitney, D. and Yager, T. (eds.) (2000). *Appreciative Inquiry: Rethinking human organization toward a positive theory of change.* Champaign, IL: Stipes Publishing.

Melnick, J. and Roos, S. (2007). 'The myth of closure', *Gestalt Review,* 11(2), pp. 90–107.

Melnick, J. and Nevis, E. (eds.) (2012). *Mending the world: social healing interventions by Gestalt practitioners worldwide.* New York: Routledge (Taylor & Francis).

Melnick J. and Nevis, S. (1987). 'Power, choice and surprise', *The Gestalt Journal,* 9, pp. 43-51.

Melnick, J. and Nevis, S. (2016). 'Optimism', G*estalt Review,* 21(3), pp. 191-199.

Melnick, J. and Nevis S. (2018) *The Evolution of the Cape Cod Model: Gestalt Conversations, Theory and Practice.* Massachusetts: Gestalt International Study Center, Italy: Institut di Gestalt HCC.

Nevis, E. (1987). *Organizational Consulting: A Gestalt approach.* New York: Gardner Press.

Nevis, E., Melnick, J. and Nevis, S. (2008). 'Organizational change through powerful micro-level interventions: The Cape Cod Model', *OD Practitioner,* 3(40), pp. 4-8.

Perls, F. Hefferline, R. and Goodman, P. (1951). *Gestalt therapy: Excitement and growth in the human personality.* New York: Julian Press.

Chapter 12: Gestalt Practice in Large Complex Social Systems: Communities, Clans, Tribes and Other Collective Cultural Configurations

Chantelle Wyley

Gestalt theory began with research into the psychology of individual perception, and proceeded with a therapeutic approach based on individual awareness-raising and choice expansion. Soon the approach was applied within families, and groups and organizations. Much of this theory and practice development took place in Western Europe and the United States. With the advent of international Gestalt organization development programs, the Gestalt approach was applied to large social systems, including socio-economic development contexts, especially in Africa.

In collectivist Africa (as well as Asia and the Middle East) interest, motivation, obligation and relationships function differently from those in the individualistic United States and Western Europe. In African societies people identify with group needs and interests, and family and social life are deeply influenced by communal, clan and tribal connections and obligations. Western cultures enshrine individual rights, and work ethics in society and organizations value individual goal orientation, outcomes, responsibility and agency.

Gestalt practice encountered tension with eliciting an "I want" in these predominately "We need" cultures. This chapter explores how Gestalt has been applied in cultural contexts where collectivism is the defining principle informing identity and interaction and enquires whether an individualized sense of self is necessary for Gestalt to have impact.

Collectivist values and beliefs in African culture are outlined, supported by theories of cultural difference that define the individualism-collectivism polarity. Gestalt's application and applicability in collective and communal cultural contexts, is described drawing on a personal history of international Gestalt organization development and leadership programs, and applying Gestalt in Africa.

Gestalt Practice: The Individual and the Collective

Gestalt theory began with investigations into the psychology of individual perception at the Berlin Psychological Institute after World War I. This work was applied in individual psychotherapy by Fritz and Laura Perls, Paul Goodman and others, from the 1930s. Even with the focus on individual experience these early researchers and therapists were interested in the collective. In Berlin, Wolfgang Köhler, Max Wertheimer, Kurt Koffka, Kurt Lewin, Bluma Zeigarnik and others explored individual perception and behavior in the context of circumstances, environment, and the whole. They were shaped by the tumultuous, emergent, modern world, two World Wars, anti-Semitism, and the rise and fall of Fascism.

Lewin's field theory considered helpful and hindering forces in society; his theories of leadership were the first to consider relational aspects of leading and following. The Perls's approach to therapy departed from Freudian historical exploration of individual psyches, and engaged with patient-therapist dynamics in current experience. They were clear about the wider implications of individual awareness-raising and choice expansion: a better world would result from more healthily functioning individuals. Socially conscious, they saw psychotherapy as social activism. The individuals was considered in communal contexts, but remained the focus of intervention and therapy.

In the 1950s and '60s Gestalt expanded its skill base to work with couples, families and intimate systems, and by the 1980s was including task-oriented systems in organizations (Nevis, 1987). In 1978 the Gestalt Institute of Cleveland launched its Organization and Systems Development (OSD) program, followed by an international program (the IOSD) in 1993, with a strong emphasis on intercultural contact (Rainey Tolbert, 2014). Unlike mechanical models of organization development (OD) Gestalt retained its humanistic intent and commitment, supporting healthy relational functioning in leaders and teams, with the collective and the culture as context.

The large social systems context made demands on Gestalt OD. Training programs attracted participants who sought to apply Gestalt to social change and socio-economic development. In 1995–6, a group of development practitioners joined the IOSD program in search of an approach to group dynamics, power, leadership-followership, and intercultural communication that would support and complement development planning, especially in Africa (Lohmeier and Wyley, 2009). Jochen

Lohmeier, a German economic geographer who had spent two decades in Africa, and John Nkum, a regional planner from Ghana, led this initiative. They were joined by Nathaniel Mjema, a regional planner from Tanzania, and this author, a community development worker from South Africa. They recruited participants who work in government and development in Africa to the IOSD, and later its successor, the International Gestalt Organization and Leadership Development (iGOLD) program. The program responded by extending its content to address large systems change, and by recruiting African faculty (Nkum and this author) working in socio-economic development rather than traditional OD.

The contexts in which these participants and faculty applied Gestalt were different, economically, socially, politically and culturally from the contexts of United States-based faculty and Western Gestalt OD practitioners. Development projects and programs involve wide groups of stakeholders with different governance systems, and seldom operate with clear hierarchies or accountabilities like most businesses or corporate organizations. Results are not measured in numbers or profit, but in social benefits. A key difference was how interest, motivation, obligation and relationships function in Africa, and much of Asia and the Middle East. The United States and Western Europe are characterized by individualism, with individual rights enshrined, and work ethics in society and organizations valuing individual goal orientation, outcomes, responsibility and agency. In contrast, African society is collective and communal, with people identifying with group needs and interests, and family and social life are still deeply influenced by clan and tribal connections and obligations.

Gestalt Theory: The Individual Focus

The biological model of O/E – organism in an interdependent relationship with its environment – was considered from a psychological perspective by researchers at the Berlin Institute. They observed the primal tendency of the individual (O) to complete rapidly the incomplete, create wholes based on previous experience or need, in processing environmental (E) stimuli. This process of figure formation from environmental ground formed the basis for understanding human behavior. The context is a complex field of other persons and systems, collectives and cultures, historical relationships and experiences, memories, habits, patterns of interaction.

Gestalt psychologists identified the primary organism/environment contact as motivated by need. Individual need in the moment or derived from experience fuels engagement across the contact boundary with others. Clarity and health proceed from awareness of the need and possibilities for meeting that need, given the resources of the environment. This frame has been supported by modern neuroscience – neuropsychoanalyst Mark Solms asserts "the job of the mind is to mediate between the internal world with ever-present needs, and the external world which can potentially fulfil our needs, but which is indifferent to us" (Solms, 2016).

Gestalt therapy offers in-the-moment awareness-raising that expands the individual's choices of behaviors and responses to the environment, using the therapeutic context to experiment with different perception possibilities and experiences. The Gestalt Cycle of Experience dissects and slows down the process of human experience, enabling attention to sensory stimuli, awareness expansion, choice for action, contact, and fuller experience of self and others. Gestalt therapy uses the construct of a boundary to support the individual's definition in the environment, the separation of the "me" and the "not-me", as a starting point for working with sensation and awareness, and contacting others at the boundary. A separated, individualistic sense of self with clear boundaries is implicit in Gestalt's understanding of experience and therapeutic work to enhance experience. Fritz Perls' s Gestalt prayer is a strong confirmation of this:

> "I do my thing. You do your thing. I am not in this world to live up to your expectations. And you are not in this world to live up to mine. You are you and I am I. And if by chance we find each other; it's beautiful. If not, it can't be helped."
> (Perls, 1969, p. 4)

From this stance questions may arise as to whether the Gestalt emphasis on individualized boundaries (clarification and establishment) is/should always be the focal point of Gestalt intervention, and if an individualized sense of self is required for Gestalt to have impact? How has Gestalt been applied in cultural contexts where collectivism rather, is a defining principle of identity and social interaction?"

The African Experience: A Collective Context

A key concept in African philosophy is that of *Ubuntu*, the idea that a person exists in a collective: "*Umuntu nguMuntu ngabantu*" means "A person is a person because of others"; it is also translated as "I am because you are, we are because you are" (Khoza, 2018). In Africa *every child is my child*. The slogan of the South Africa Congress of Trade Unions throughout the anti-apartheid struggle was "An injury to one is an injury to all".

> "*Ubuntu* is both a philosophy of life and a worldview. It is a comprehensive mode through which reality is constructed and shared" (Khoza, 2018).

In African culture boundaries between individuals are not explicit or primary in social bonds and engagements. Rather, extended families and clans or tribal allegiances are reference points for understanding social dynamics. Decision making in traditional African contexts takes place collectively in a consultative forum (known in South Africa as a *lekgotla*, from the Sotho or Tswana word for courtyard); here circular inputs and sharing, highly respectful of the whole, take place. Communication depends on subtleties and involves complex sub-texts relating to the relationships between sender and receiver and their extended families. With strong oral traditions and connections over generations, explicit and written documentation is unnecessary and decisions are taken communally with witnesses and networks ensuring commitment (Meyer, 2014, pp. 31, 58). Ownership of resources is collective among extended families and clans, and in villages and settlements boundaries between fields and homesteads may not be fixed or delineated. The identity of the individual is derived from the group, to which the individual owes loyalty based on practical and psychological dependence: the group is the source of protection against life's hardships (Hofstede, 1997, p. 50–52). In cases where individuals need to be singled out (disciplined, praised) this is done in a way that maintains harmony and the integrity of the group (praise is not too distinctive, and discipline involves obligations to others and evokes fear of rejection). Personal opinions that differ from the group are rarely expressed, even formulated, as individuals take their bearings from others, mainly elders and tradition.

African collective identity and obligation extends powerfully into the modern Westernized world of work. African professionals working in the skyscrapers of Johannesburg take care of dependent relatives. They educate the children of siblings, fund unemployed uncles, build houses for older relatives, as part of what is referred to as "Black tax". This practice is unquestioned and accepted; it's the way things are "supposed to be" (Personal communications). Service to the extended family is expected and is respected as a social contribution. It is part of who and what it means to be African. In the culture of the Xhosa people an incoming daughter-in-law is renamed by her senior in-laws, with a name that indicates her value to the family (Personal communication).

The application of Gestalt in the context of collective culture was a point of discussion for this author and colleagues involved in facilitating development projects and programs, funded by German development co-operation.* Central to our work was a six week program in development management at which development managers from African, Asian and Middle Eastern countries met in Berlin. The cultural differences were stark and alive.

To support us in intercultural management and communication we used Dutch anthropologist Geert Hofstede's research into dimensions of cultural difference (1997), and we included his framework and self-questionnaire in the program content. This raised awareness of our cultural assumptions and those of others. Individualism-collectivism was the area with most extreme differences between Africa (scores of 20–27), Asian countries (scores in the 40s), Arab states (scores in the 30s), and the United States (score of 91) and most of Western Europe (high 60s to 80s). Power distance was also a notable area of difference between high Africa and low Europe/US. In dialogues around individualism–collectivism we noted differences regarding sense of self/identity (based on personal self versus part of a group), belonging (loose connections between individuals versus strong cohesion in groups), care (look after self and close nuclear family versus be protected by the extended family group in exchange for loyalty), interest (self-interest versus group interest), ownership (resources accumulated by individuals versus shared and distributed among relatives), quality of life (personal freedom and individual development versus being cared for and protected by others), work relationships (clear business and contracts versus mutual obligations with gifts and favoritism), communication (open, direct, confronting messaging versus social harmony and saving

---

* The German Foundation for International Development (DSE), later Capacity Building International (InWEnt), offered training and capacity building support to German-funded projects and programs supported via German Technical Cooperation (GTZ).

face with indirect communication), and independence or interdependence. The difference between individualistic Germans and collectivist Africans and Asians was marked.

As a white English-speaking South African with Protestant Scottish and English ancestry, this author has individualistic tendencies typical of cultures with pioneering settler histories, also socially unconventional (Hofstede, 1991, p.77; Sapolsky, 2017, p. 277; Meyer, 2014, p.129). Mixed with this came five generations in rural Africa, and the family's strong sense of connection with others, responsibility for others, obligation, consideration, charity / service. Apartheid paternalism and oppression also defined a sense of difference and complex interdependence and survival among and across races. Hofstede's definition of bi-cultural individuals, susceptible to cultural clues and able to process stimuli differently depending on context (Hofstede, 1997, p.277) resonates.

African colleagues close to their traditional roots lived the tension between individualism and collectivism. One colleague's father had numerous wives and 40 children of which he was the eldest son. Educated in the early years of African independence he attained a master's degree at a German university. He identified as a Christian and founded a successful consulting firm, representing a break from the tribal, clan and collective culture of his parents' generation. And, in our work together we witnessed the tension between his respectful obligations to extended family and clan, and providing education and financial security for his nuclear family.

In 2016 in a leadership seminar with senior African public sector auditors, discussions focused on African leaders' challenges in stepping up to lead. The discussion identified the tension between collectivist obligations to others in traditional African culture and Western individualism and accountability. One senior official exclaimed

> "That's it! I feel I am two people: one in the office and a different one when I go home. I think I am going mad sometimes, reconciling the two!" (Personal communication).

The discussion increased awareness of the personally experienced individualist-collectivist tension, and the behavioral contradictions in social and work existences. Acceptance and ownership of the tension brought a sense of integration and wholeness.

Gestalt Interventions: The Application of Gestalt in a Collective Cultural Context

In 2011–2013 a team of us worked on a culture change program in a provincial government in South Africa. At a particularly frustrating point in the two year process, a senior official partnering our team, exclaimed:

> "We won't be able to get anything done or change anything in this province, until people stop referring to each other by their clan names!" (Personal communication).

Culture has been described by Robert Sapolsky (Sapolsky, 2017) as a key influence on human behavior-in-the-moment, along with the brain (systems prioritizing survival and connection), hormones (chemical (im) balances), genetics, and childhood experiences (many of which are culturally determined). Together these influences override rational, strategic, in-the-moment responses to another person, group or situation.

In our change program, we explored whether Gestalt could be used to raise awareness of cultural assumptions about clan obligations, the dominance of the group, leaders not standing out or shaming others, and deep social interdependence? The province was crying out for exceptional leadership as clinics and hospitals, schools and the police system failed citizens, especially the poor.

The design of the culture change program was developed by Gestalt-trained consultants contracted by the South African National Treasury's Technical Assistance Unit (TAU), supported by the Teleos Leadership Institute (Philadelphia, USA)*, specialists in leadership development in service of resonant and productive workplaces.

The data collection was conducted together with internal change agents using an appreciative inquiry-derived tool, Dynamic Inquiry (London and McMillen, 1992). From close to 300 interviews, the following themes emerged, confirming that collective cohesion was valued above achievement and results:

1 Developing relationships in the spirit of *Batho Pele* (People First)[†] needs to occur at all levels of government.

---

* The TAU team was led by this author; Teleos consultants were Annie McKee, Fran Johnston, Eddy Mwelwa. See www.teleosleers.com
† *Batho Pele* (Sotho for "people first") is a South African government initiative to improve quality and accessibility of government services, with a focus on public good.

2   Communication norms point to widespread distress in the organisational culture, leading to isolation, frustration, low morale, and ultimately, ineffective service delivery.
3   We hunger for a strong and transparent leadership.
4   We must confront the multiple issues contributing to poor performance.
5   Favoritism, special interest groups, and political posturing make it difficult to ensure quality service delivery.
6   The limited availability of even the most basic resources is a barrier to effective job performance.
7   Promised but undelivered human resources puts too much stress on me and my team.
8   I am motivated to excel at service delivery, but my peers hold me back.
(Lohmeier, Mwelwa, and Wyley, 2013, p21)

These themes point to high awareness of collectivist assumptions and priorities, preventing fairness and merit from flourishing in the public service. At the same time they show yearning for togetherness, conformity and safety and care in and for the group. Notice the use of the passive voice, and preponderance of large system issues suggesting own helplessness. Theme 8 shows how any positive individualism in service of the people of the province, is dealt with cruelly.

The diagnostic report also identified meta-themes; again these illustrate I–we tension:
- We, public servants of the [province], know what will work.
- We blame our leaders, without ourselves owning that we can influence people.
- We do not take personal responsibility as much as we could.
- We are passionate about *Batho Pele* and all its principles and philosophies.
- There is profound confusion about what it really means to be a leader.

(Lohmeier, Mwelwa, and Wyley, 2013, p21)

The cultural differences between consultants and provincial officials needed careful management. Workshop facilitation focused on affirmation and acknowledgment, establishment of belonging among change agents, and inspirational and optimistic messaging, together with an emphasis on responsibility and the officials' ownership of the process. From the outset our team worked with the assumption that:

> "If the change agents were to take on the role of driving the culture change initiative throughout the province, it was essential that they develop relational leadership skills (resonant leadership) that would enable them *to own fully their individual responsibilities* in driving the change."
> (Author's italics). (Lohmeier, Mwelwa, and Wyley, 2013, p.12)

An emotional intelligence leadership program over three days enabled optimistic group cohesion and spirit, intertwined with individual self-reflection and ownership of own behavior, through sharing and storytelling of life histories and experiences in small groups. Contact in the large group was nurtured with facilitation that kept respectfully on the boundary of their process, avoiding an expert consulting presence, but with enough authority to provide safety. The consultants fostered relationships of mutual acceptance and care with the change agents, using empathy and challenge, with far less differentiation than in more individualistic contexts

The program ended its first phase in March 2013. A case study report[*] reflected participants' significant personal learning: self-awareness, as well as insights into change management, leadership, skill in culture research, influencing, and working in teams. An amalgamation of responses illustrates individuation:

> "I am more... able to deal with my emotions, my self-management, being more assertive, confident,... restrain from reacting in a negative environment even at home, I learnt to be patient, have empathy...I discovered my strengths and weaknesses ...I contain and manage my emotions, voicing out ill feelings without being confrontational, self-awareness, talking less and listening more (Lohmeier, Mwelwa and Wyley, 2013, pp. 51–52).

The case study noted the consultants' ability to use their presence:

> This program offered a type of leadership to the change agent group that adhered to the Gestalt approach of offering a *consulting presence* (Rainey and Hanafin, 2006) lacking in the client system...The facilitation team... offered...an experience of supportive leadership, building capacity and facilitating individual and systems development. This deliberate use of self gave the change

---

[*] Lohmeier, Mwelwa and Wyley, 2013

agents an experience of leadership that evoked own power and agency, as well as a different definition of followership. This was a design and intention of the delivery of the program, and is unique in its deliberateness and prominence among TAU projects (Lohmeier, Mwelwa and Wyley, 2013, p. 32).

The specific approach, to work with the individual change agent's awareness and sense of self was commented on as follows:

> The central design premise of the program – that of *intervening at an intra-personal level with individuals* in the interests of system change – was found to be remarkably successful... Evaluation forms from the various sessions of the training attest to the shifts in individuals as do self reports on the impact of behavior change on their teams and other work place systems (Lohmeier, Mwelwa and Wyley, 2013, p. 32–33).

The approach directly worked with underlying assumptions and drivers of behavior; something unique in a government intervention in South Africa:

> [The provincial government] officials... operate in *large beyond-organisation systems*, where there is not a 'one power hierarchy', but a mix of political and institutional powers... Decisions are made by a variety of individuals, sub-groups, groups, and organisations with different motivations, interests and affiliations. Some of the strongest and most influential motivators are sub-conscious... Programs like this one that seek to influence this 'field' with regard to the behaviour of individuals and groups, and to influence the drivers of behaviour, require special attention to field attractors and special approaches for complexity and emergence (Lohmeier, Mwelwa and Wyley, 2013, p. 33).

Gestalt Learnings and Adaptations

Gestalt work, in the service of wholeness, focusses on integration of alienated parts of a system or the self. Our work in African collective cultures involves not a choice between individual or collective approaches, but client support that navigates and integrates both. The contact boundaries of both the individual and the collective deserve respect and attention. Our clients already live in both worlds, managing tension between cultural assumptions and obligations and the need to respect backgrounds and traditions, and the demands of the individualistic world of work in which they seek personal recognition and success.

Working in collective cultures requires more intensive joining on the part of the intervener than in individualistic contexts. Building relationships with clients and acceptance by the group is the essence of entry and contracting work in such systems. In this author's case, as a white woman working for African government clients in the context of recent oppression, this required time and sensitivity. Part of this process requires the use of "we" language, and "us" and "together", creating acceptance and belonging between clients and consultant.

In the provincial government program, providing a presence which the (harsh, hierarchical, collectivist, government) client system lacked, necessitated working with acknowledgment, affirmation, generosity, respect and love. An inability to speak the local language was not necessarily an impediment; what was important was the intentional, subtle, emotional communications that accompanied messages.

In good Gestalt practice initial joining requires eventual differentiating for learning to take place. In this context, suggested individualistic stances that would disrupt cultural assumptions that were stifling service delivery, were communicated in an unthreatening way. This contrasted with the menacing tone of usual messages from national government officials and technical advisers. In this way an individualistic presence was attractively offered; and this model encouraged change agents to experiment with their own behavioral range.

Knowing that a deep need for connection and safety and group identity exists with African (and Asian and Arab) participants, helped us to understand informal African sub-group formations in our international learning programs. We saw this fulfilling a need to create a sense of family, of home. Hofstede refers to the need for in-group–outgroup distinction being high in collectivist cultures and a tendency for participants on learning programs to gravitate towards faculty from the same backgrounds, requesting special connections or preferential treatment or more support (Hofstede, 1997, p.62). This has been the case with South African and Ghanaian participants and respective IOSD and iGOLD faculty members, who balance care while effecting distance in their faculty presence.

In group learning in collective cultures, it is our experience that the separation between self and others may need to be introduced carefully. Along with building a relationship between the facilitator and the group, and a sense of belonging and connection, workshop openings need solid grounding in purpose and rationale and the benefit of the work for a wider group. This needs not to be merely stated, but affirmed with particular meaning until there is a felt sense of mission in the group, especially where African government platitudes about "service delivery to our people" have become hollow and meaningless. In personal group work and team coaching sessions, inviting opening statements of "I want…" and "we need…" may require switching order and inviting "we need…" and "I want…" In general, people from collective cultures may favor small group work, since speaking up in large groups where affiliations are not clear or established, may be unfamiliar.

In African culture, communal stories and narratives preserve and sustain identities, and create a sense of belonging. Inviting the sharing of stories, legends, proverbs and wisdom in a learning or work group is familiar and has impact in collective cultures. In the provincial change program, after discussing the interview themes, we invited change agents to envisage the future. In circles seated on the floor they were invited to share dreams, as grandparents share stories – this explicitly evoked African fireside story-telling.*

Closing

In the modern and modernizing Africa of today, both the collectivistic and individualistic worlds exist. Naming and attending to this tension, as with all polarities, has merit, bringing awareness and integration, relief and satisfaction.

At the time of his research (1980s) Hofstede identified a correlation between a country's wealth and individualism (Hofstede, 1987 p.53). He suggested that countries with collectivist cultures that were moving toward more individualism would support wealth creation and create opportunities to move out of poverty. This may point to the importance of supporting young Africans to individuate, and step into a "modern" identity.

---

* Annie McKee, Teleos Leadership Institute and IOSD graduate, has credit for the design and facilitation of this session.

However, Hofstede also noted the increasing significance and success in the world economy of collectivist Eastern cultures, and he commented on the declining care for the aged in Japan as the population becomes wealthier and as interests become more individual (Hofstede, 1997, p.77). Yet concern for the collective remains a cultural priority. Singapore government programs emphasize care and support for citizens (community health days, maids-day-off campaigns) amidst flourishing individual wealth creation.

At the top of the individualism scale, the United States over the past 20 years has shown a swing towards management and leadership practices that focus on people and relationships – on emotional intelligence for example (Goleman, Boyatzis and McKee, 2001). Approaches to intimacy, for example "love languages" (Chapman and White, 2011) and parent-child frameworks in transactional analysis, are being used in the workplace with success. At a global level the integration of individualism and collectivism seems to be happening, with aspects of both having the possibility of contributing to an increase in wealth and sustainability (sharing of wealth across populations).

This chapter explores whether the individual contact boundary is necessarily the focus of Gestalt work in collective cultures. Our experience is that the individual self, in the African collective context today, is highly receptive to attention and support, and the response to this support, when elegantly and sensitively offered and administered, is one of appreciation and relief.

Sapolsky, in a stirring piece on humans' primal tendency to sort into Us–Them and judge accordingly, urges us to slow ourselves down to "individuate, individuate, individuate" (Sapolsky, 2017, p.387–424). The tendency to automaticity in our behavior requires individual boundary and awareness work to enable choice and change.

Our reflections about contact in collective cultures has taught us that the individual is not always the starting point, nor is an individualized sense of self necessary for Gestalt to have impact. Collective cultures define themselves around in-group behavior, and working in and with these assumptions requires a clear stance of joining as a fellow human being, whilst still holding the stance of a change agent, at the boundary of difference offering potential for change and growth.

References:

Chapman, G. and White, P. (2011). *The 5 Languages of Appreciation in the Workplace*. Chicago: Northfield.

Goleman, D., Boyatzis, R. and McKee, A. (2001). *Primal Leadership: realizing the power of emotional intelligence*. Boston: Harvard Business Publishing.

Hofstede, G. (1997). *Cultures and organizations: software of the mind*. Revised ed. New York: McGraw-Hill.

Khoza, R. (2018). *Concepts of Ubuntu and attuned leadership*. Address, 17 February 2018. [online] http://www.reuelkhoza.co.za/reuelkhoza/wp-content/uploads/2018/06/Concepts-of-Ubuntu-Attuned-Leadership2018.pdf. (Accessed: 10 December 2018)

Lohmeier, J. and Wyley, C. (2009). 'Using Gestalt methods in training managers of development projects and programs in developing countries' in Melnick, J. and Nevis, E.C. (eds.) *Mending the world: social healing interventions by Gestalt practitioners worldwide*, South Wellfleet, MA: Gestalt International Study Centre, pp. 241--263.

Lohmeier, J., Mwelwa, E. and Wyley, C. (2013). *Case study: Culture Change Program*. Pretoria: National Treasury, Technical Assistance Unit. [unpublished]

London, A. and McMillen, M. C. (1992). 'Discovering social issues: organization development in a multi-cultural community' *Journal of Applied Behavioral Science* 28(3), pp. 445–460.

Nevis, E.C. (1987). *Organizational consulting: a Gestalt approach*. Cleveland: Gestalt Institute of Cleveland Press.

Meyer, E. (2014). *The Culture Map: decoding how people think, lead, and get things done across cultures*. New York: PublicAffairs.

Perls, F. (1969). *Gestalt therapy verbatim*. Lafayette, Ca: Real People Press.

Rainey Tolbert, M. A. (2014). 'What is Gestalt organization and systems development? All about the O, the S, the D…and of course, Gestalt' *OD practitioner* 36(4), pp. 6–10.

Rainey Tolbert, M. A. and Hanafin. J. (2006). 'Use of self in organizational consulting: what matters is presence' in Jones, B. and Brazzal, M. (eds.) *The NTL Handbook of organization development and change: principles, practice and perspectives*. San Francisco: Pfeiffer, pp. 69–82.

Sapolsky, R. (2017). *Behave: the biology of humans at our best and worst*. London: Bodley Head.

Solms, M. (2015). *The Feeling Brain*. London: Karnac.

Solms, M. (2016). [Personal communication in online course, "What is a mind?"] University of Cape Town and FutureLearn.

Chapter 13: Case Study: A Holistic Strategy to Promote Change in a Multinational Corporation

Eugenio Molini

I have been working on-and-off since 2010, and very actively during the last two years, with a multinational corporation whose business is to develop and deliver learning products and services to educational institutions. My assignment is to support its movement from operating as a hierarchical, vertically structured organization, towards operating in a more holistic interconnected mode.

I acquired the Gestalt approach in my trainings, in the 1980's as therapist and in the 1990's as OD-consultant. To Gestalt I owe the ground I stand on when I work and live. During many years I have meditated about what Gestalt means for me beyond the theories and methods. And this is what I have understood (Figure 1: Gestalt).

1. Gestalt is firstly a philosophy that successfully explains life at the fringes of the mystery of existence, without ever attempting to explain the mystery itself.
2. Gestalt is secondly a personal practice to intentionally approach, embrace and experience the mystery, without ever fully understanding it.
3. Gestalt is thirdly a professional practice that allows us to support others (people, organizations, communities …) to be what they are and do what they do in the field that has the mystery at its center.

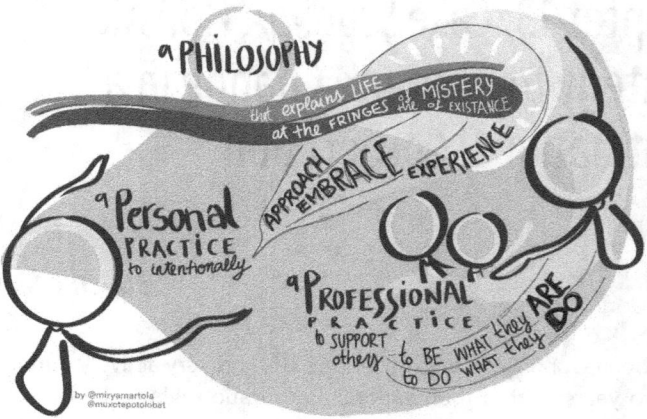

Figure 1: Gestalt

But the pain of not understanding the mystery can be so deep and intense! I needed to have some comfort somewhere, and I found it in the Systemic approach, that allows me to put myself in a meta-position towards what is going on, including my own experience. It is also a great comfort for my clients when I come up with a Systemic explanation of what is going on.

Comforting as this may be, the Gestalt approach is the trump card that makes everything come into place, as everything starts and ends in the experience of the mystery of existence, in contact with others that also connect with it.

The dilemma between pure experience of life at the fringes of the mystery and the need to understand, permeates my approach and the concepts I use in my work. You will see the dilemma in the case description. You will see it in the fact that the case description itself is a systemic description of something that can only be understood when experienced. Finally, you will see it in the concepts I share at the end of the article.

CHAPTER 13: CASE STUDY: A HOLISTIC STRATEGY TO PROMOTE CHANGE IN A MULTINATIONAL CORPORATION

Case Description

When I design change processes, or I give feedback on a design as it is the case here, I tend to accept the What of the proposed change as a given.

My contribution is to work towards a design that integrates How, Who, and When, aligned towards the client's desired future.

It is from this perspective that I gave my input 2011

2011 Prequel

The initiation of this transformational process was clearly adaptive. During years, the Corporation as a whole, and the companies that formed it, responded to sociological, technological and environmental changes with a multitude of decisions. Each decision was sound in itself and didn't affect greatly the Corporation as a whole, but as they imperceptibly accumulated, they triggered internal and external tensions.

Some strategical visionaries at Business Intelligence began to detect these tensions early on. Reality would confirm some years later that they correctly interpreted the signs as a forewarning of a still unspecified risk of becoming obsolete in a not so far future. A sense of urgency compelled them to prematurely elaborate a change plan. 2011, the team that elaborated this plan consulted me on its design, before they presented it to the Corporate Management Team (CMT).

My response 2011 was that their plan was elegantly conceived, but that it would have little positive impact and probably much negative. Without commenting the what of the change My feedback on the plan was as follows:
- The plan depicted a bright future, implicitly sent the message that everything that had been done up to the moment was wrong.
- The plan focused on the What mostly. But the proposed Who, When and How followed the traditional cascading procedure, at odds with the idea of one aspect of the What: getting away from the silo-organization and moving towards a more interconnected organization.

- The plan would most probably awaken resistances directed towards the How, even in cases in which co-workers and mid-managers agreed with the What. In the end the change process would stall, leaving in its wake a lot of hurt people, disintegrated units and organizational weariness, without any movement forward to show.
- The plan acknowledged the most predictable resistances, those directed towards the What of the proposed change. The plan didn't consider adequately other forces that would work against the proposed change, such as:
  - the loss of control that mid-managers would suffer;
  - the investment that had been done along the years on developing procedures and best practices;
  - the affiliations and loyalties among people that had worked together for a long time;
- The What of the change was primarily defined by a conception of Digital Transformation that emphasized the digital aspects (IT, Systems, Communication, etc.) and not so much the transformational aspects (People, Organization, Business Model, etc.)
- The plan was responsive to perceived threats, but I could see that that the brilliant future it depicted would eventually clash with the Corporation's current mission.
- I couldn't see that the plan allowed for a way of promoting the desired change in a way that was congruent at different organizational scales (organization as a whole, business unit, team, individual) and in different time scales (strategic time, project time, meeting time.)

The 2011 plan was an immature first glimpse of what was to come five years later. I have no idea about what happened with that plan. Some good impression must my feedback have made, because 2016, I was engaged to work on the real thing.

2011 – 2016 Interval

By 2016, when I was contacted me for the second time, the Corporation had done a lot of work. Four aspects are most relevant:
1. Based on a thorough analysis, the Corporation had formulated a consistent hypothesis of what was going on;
2. They had formulated a vison of what the Corporation needed to become;

3. Considering 1 and 2, they had re-formulated their mission.
4. Instead of developing a linear cascading change plan, they had developed an adaptive Transformation process design. The most relevant differences between both ways of promoting change are:

	Adaptive design	**Linear plan**
Departure	Accept that multiple points of departure. The different Business Units, teams, stakeholders in the value-chain and Individuals start from different points.	Much time and effort are invested in bringing stakeholders to the same base camp, before they can move together in coordinated action.
Direction / Goal	Multiple stakeholders move towards a horizon that looks different from different points in the organization and moves as we move.	Change is conceived as climbing a mountain, whose top is fixed and doesn't change. All stakeholders should move together and look at the top from the same place.
Governance	Governed by systemic non-linear guidelines for adaptive action in complex systems.	Governed by either/or rules and linear procedures with the intention of controlling the complex process.
How	Each step is congruent with the desired future.	Each step is congruent with the plan.
Who	Whoever can contribute to address an issue or take a step is welcome.	Whoever has responsibility within the vertical organization or transversal projects or processes.
What	A desired future that evolves as the organization moves towards it.	Predefined in the plan, with KPIs and other predictors. Problem management.
Time	The way you get to the future is the future you create.	Push the organization towards the goal / top of the mountain.

2016 – Triggers

The tensions detected and the patterns they formed, were structured as four crises that the Corporate Transformation needed to address:
- **Crisis of Intensity:** people felt the pressure to work in many projects and collaborate across many organizational boundaries, with small chances of enjoying a sense of accomplishment anywhere;
- **Crisis of Complexity:** the management systems and organizational structure had become cumbersome, and were perceived as inadequate for the current level of internal and external complexity;
- **Crisis of Adjustment:** maladjustment with the external reality, mostly in technology, but also in sociological and environmental issues.
- **Crisis of Growth:** slowdown of the company's overall rate of growth and a decrease in profitability in some of their more mature markets.

2016 – A new mission

The mission statement that needed to be revised was: We deliver high quality products to education and culture institutions so that they can fulfill their mission.

The new holistic mission became: We contribute to the development of whole persons and to the humanistic transformation of society by delivering high quality products and services to education and culture.

The difference between the two mission statements shows clearly the direction in which the company needed to move in order to achieve the desired holistic transformation.

2016 and ongoing:

When I was contacted 2016, the new mission had already been defined. The work on the mission had helped those involved to see that the Company would not address the four crises identified earlier if it conceived the change process linearly, as climbing the mountain of the Digital Transformation. The insight was there that the Company needed to move holistically towards a holistic horizon, being the development of their Digital Business a key sector of that horizon.

CHAPTER 13: CASE STUDY: A HOLISTIC STRATEGY TO PROMOTE CHANGE IN A MULTINATIONAL CORPORATION

This time, the client and I formulated my assignment as supporting the emergence of an informal Network of Promoters **(the Who)** of a new way of working that addressed the four Crises **(the What)** in a way that was congruent with the mission **(The How)**.

People were invited to the Network of Promoters following three criteria:

1. **How favorable they are to the proposed change.** If you want to build critical mass in the organization, you don't want a Network of Promoters formed by only enthusiasts. That would be a hallelujah group with no impact whatsoever. You want to invite enthusiasts and people who have some resistance to the proposed change. You neither want to have in the Network of Promoters people that are overly comfortable in the organizational inertias or too resistant. The risk then is that the network becomes a pressure cooker whose main occupation is to convince the late adopters and those who are immune to change, instead of building critical mass.

2. **How well connected and informally influential they are.** If you want to avoid a traditional cascade model and use a dissemination mode, you want to invite people that are connected to many people across vertical and horizontal organizational boundaries. You want them also to be influential because of the trust their connections deposit in them. The well connected and those who are enthusiastic will most probably not be the same people. It is good that the well-connected have some kind of resistance to the proposed change. Their influence depends a lot in the trust deposited in them, and the trust depends on their ability to relate to what their connections are concerned about.

3. **The formal position they have in the structure.** If you want to draw on the power of hierarchy, you need that the people with real formal power in the organization support the Network of Promoters. But you don't want to have too big power differences among the people invited to the Network of Promoters. Typically, the best is to invite middle managers from two different hierarchical levels. Exceptions should be made for those co-workers that, by virtue of their knowledge and experience, enjoy high prestige among middle management and are not easily "power stricken".

Non-linear guidelines for How to promote adaptive change

The Network of Promoters, having understood that **the How needed to be congruent with the What**, developed Guidelines for How to promote the Transformation:
1. Promote change by building critical mass across vertical and horizontal organizational boundaries, aiming initially towards **diminishing organizational inertias. Acknowledge resistances** as they emerge, collaborating with them as **loyal forces for continuity** that express what different players and parts of the organization think is **important to keep.** Discern when and where some **inertias** need to be actively engaged, giving them the opportunity to become conscious resistances directed to the **What**.
2. Promote change as **a fractal process in non-linear time**, by designing each activity as an experience of solving the issues that currently concern those involved, using prototypes of the new way of working. This is an example of how to bring the desired future to the present instead of pushing the organization towards a pre-defined goal.
3. Promote change as a **fractal process in the multilayered organizational space,** by designing each activity as a prototype of the new way of working, offering the participants the experience of solving today's issues by collaborating in autonomous and interdependent teams across multiple organizational boundaries.

Commu-Nety of Practice (Community + Network)

The Network of Promoters meet regularly in a format we call Commu-Nety of Practice CoP, which is a recurring one-day session, open for all the promoters who can/want to attend. The purpose is to support each other to promote change with the most impact regarding the **What**, and the least pain for people (including themselves), as well as minimizing the wear-and-tear in the organization. This ambition is congruent with the mission of the Company.

The CoP sessions are centered on Case-Work. A Case is any current change situation, project, assignment, etc. in which a promoter is excited, challenged or frustrated, and in a position to influence.

Each participant in a CoP session has the opportunity to present a case. Following the Case-work procedure, the rest support the case-owner, practice interdependent leadership and apply a systemic approach. Each promoter retains responsibility for the case he/she presents, and at the same time receives input from all the others. The Networked Promoters don't need to agree on how to go about change. The principles that govern the change process emerge from the work on specific cases.

Now

The emerging insight in the Network of Promoters is that the organization is getting close to the Transformation Zone (see figure above). The insight includes also the conviction that only a powerful intervention by the Group Management Team will make the difference.

The Group Management Team, who had given the mandate to promote the change but hadn't been following the work of the Network of Promoters, and a sizeable number of middle managers have become aware of the operational consequences of the transformation. Much of what initially were **inertias have become explicit resistances, allowing the promoters to engage in open dialogue with the resistors,** understood as voices that want to keep some things as they are or want something else.

One of the most intense work is being done on the loss of control that managers at all levels perceive they are suffering. The strategy of the Network of Promoters is still to **address differently the inertias and the resistances**. The emerging resistances are addressed mainly in two fashions:
1. Formal meetings, in which managers of a specific Business Unit or department meet to take formal decisions about the new way of working. The networked promoters are never invited as such, but those promoters who are managers in the specific Business Unit participate as managers.
2. Work meetings in which promoters and resistors from different parts of the organization collaborate to solve current operational challenges, attending to the new way of working and what needs to be continued. The strategic aim is still to build necessary critical mass to bring the system to a tipping point. Inertias are addressed in this same fashion.

There are signs that the field of operations of the company (their competitors, the techno-sphere and the economy of large segments of their clients) is approaching tipping point, that may come as a shock for the company and force it to change faster than it capable of doing with only internal efforts. Still unknown if this will be an opportunity or a threat.

It is interesting to see the ambivalence towards the network of influencers. On the one hand they are perceived by managers and some employees as menaces and their work sabotaged. On the other hand, they are admired and jeered. This ambivalence is also present within the Group Management Team.

The dice is cast. Still impossible to know how it will fall.

Some concepts I use in the case description

Multilayered Space: the way you create the organization is the organization you create

By promoting change in a way that is consistent with the organization you want to create, you introduce a **radical change at all scales of the multilayered organizational space**: the organization's internal structure; it's way of operating in its market and value chain; the way of working and collaborating across organizational units; the mindset, identities and affiliations of managers, coworkers and other stakeholders in the organization's environment of operations; ...

Non-linear Time: A different future is possible . . . here and now!

The movement implies a **radical change in the way of changing**, a transformation of the linear perception of how change happens over time. It's no longer about pushing the organization towards the future, it's about bringing the future to the present. It's about offering to those involved opportunities to address today's issues in a manner that is congruent with the desired future. It's about accepting that for a long time, past and future will coexist in the organization's present.

Congruence across time and space

In this assignment, designing, promoting and facilitating change across a multilayered space and non-linear time means that all activities, small and big, should be congruent with the mission of the company:
- to allow those involved in each activity to be and act as whole persons
- to contribute to the humanistic transformation of the organization and its way of operating internally and externally.

Change and Continuity

The forces for change are those that push and/or pull any system in the direction of the new. **The forces for continuity** are those that compel any system to stay the same. Forces for change and forces for continuity come in several modes.

The forces for change and the forces for continuity **interact with each other within any scale of system, and between multiple scales of system**: individual, relational, group, project, organization, field of operations, society, global, planetary, …

Forces for change	Forces for continuity
Adaptation.	**Homeostasis**
Organizations respond to internal and external events with a multitude of small decisions, aiming towards changing so that nothing essential changes really. Paradoxically, the small changes accumulate imperceptibly, leading to a tipping point after which the organization deeply and irreversibly transforms.	Organizations tend to keep for as long as possible a stable and constant internal state. Homeostasis "collaborates" with Adaptation and Inertia as long as the steady internal state isn't affected.

Provoked

Sometimes, a sudden external or internal event overwhelms the organization's capacity of Homeostasis, Adaptation and Inertia, and overcomes the Resistances from stakeholders.

The organization is then brought to a tipping point after which it changes deeply and irreversibly.

Promoted

Conscious, intentional and persistent action by any stakeholder, aiming to move the organization towards a desired future.

Paradoxically, resistance is in the perception of the promoter. Those identified by the promoters as resistors see themselves as promoters of something else.

The Promoters need to be congruent in the Who, the What and the How of the change.

Learning

Learning means always that the learner, may it be an individual, a team or an organization, changes in some way.

Inertia

Organizations and people develop procedures, habits and structures that are highly resilient and promptly bring them back to business as usual.

Inertia should be differentiated from Homeostasis, as they not always point in the same direction.

Resistance

Conscious, intentional and persistent action or lack thereof, by any stakeholder who doesn't want the promoted change.

Those who are perceived by the promoters as resistors, perceive themselves often as promoters of some other change, or sometimes promoters of continuity.

The resistances can be directed towards the Who, the What and/or the How of the change.

Best practices

Best practices, however good they are, become eventually stereotypical ways of doing whatever the organization, team or individual does.

IV. GESTALT APPROACH TO CHANGE

Chapter 14: A Gestalt Approach to Optimizing Competencies During a Digital Transformation

Gudrun Frank

Similarity as Ground of Learning and Understanding Transformation

Change is constant and accelerating. It requires new, different, and differently perceptible actions. Under normal circumstances, transformations can be challenging for organizations of all sizes. Few are aware of or prepared for the challenges of transitioning to a more digital environment. Whether the shift is to new software platforms or hardware, these digital transformations require specialized and unique competencies that organizations typically do not consider. Without a Gestalt approach, these transformations could fail.

As systems enlarge and become more complexly networked, organizations often leap to incorporate technology-based solutions into their processes. These tools not only can produce spectacular and speedy results, they can be easy to use. However, their effects are often difficult to predict. If organizations misjudge the speed of change, their leap can result in missteps and undermine their objectives. To avoid this, a Gestalt approach urges them to consider what is known as ground for learning and transformation. Similarity helps them recognize and understand the speed of change. It also enables systems and individuals to respond to change more efficiently and effectively.

Similarity is also helpful when change occurs that no one really wants. This change has become their new reality and must be integrated into their everyday actions. It can be intimidating and frightening.

Individuals respond to change in a variety of ways: They can perceive it as beneficial, they can adapt to it, or they can build up great resistance against it. Whatever the reaction, they need boundaries to recognize their own competencies within the changing system. They need a tangible, measurable comparison value.

We can allay individuals' and larger systems' fears of change by helping them deliberately and responsibly leverage their own potential. Personal feedback is valuable to the process, for them and ultimately, for their companies. It supports them to consciously transcend boundaries, perceive them hopefully and act effectively.

The Gestalt Approach and Competencies

The competence of a person is defined as her or his ability to function self-responsibly and self-organized in specific situations to achieve the expected effect. This definition inspired me to develop a toolset for my consulting practice, exprobico, to determine which competencies are needed in a specific context of work or learning situation. We call it the "exprobico-check" (or probico-check). It is individually designed for every customer requirement.

The exprobico-check acknowledges that to determine a person's competencies, the consultant must know the context in which the competencies are needed. We must know the role and context in which the person or team must act, and we must know something about the cultural environment of this context. Only then we can design a landscape of the competencies and develop a benchmark for satisfying the company's requirements.

Sometimes, particularly during a digital transformation, new competencies are required. That makes it critical to determine the status quo and understand the appropriate requirements so we can consider a wide range of possibilities to develop or design these new competencies.

First, we usually build a working paper to help individuals gauge their own competencies. After they complete their competency check, it is easier for them to discover their potential, relative to the benchmark. This self-reflecting awareness is an energizing intro that enables us to successfully obtain a status quo to begin the competence development process.

It is important that clients do not assess their results independently. We immediately begin the change and the development process with personal feedback. Together, we explore the complex world of competencies.

My research has found that holistic and procedural thinking helps to find a similar solution with high complexity in the background. To fulfill the competence definition and the chance of development with practical experiences, I developed the simple structure called the "5-C Model". It consists of these elements:
- Cognition
- Can do
- Caring
- Communicating
- Cooperating

Succinctly expressed in one sentence: Anyone who is cognizant of his skills, who masters his profession and is able to thereby respond to changing environments while sharing knowledge and cooperating, requires extensive communication skills. I know that is a rather complicated sentence, so I will explore each element in the context of transformation that aims to optimize competencies. I also will offer examples of how Gestalt principles supported me in developing successful tools to address this challenge.

I drew guidance from the following Gestalt principles:
- The Level of Systems
- The Unit of work
- The Multiple Reality
- The Whole-Thinking Approach
- The Law of Prägnanz

How Gestalt Principles Correlate with the 5-C Model

Gestalt Core Concepts

Gestalt theory has inspired the development of practices that enable people to become intentional in their choices and more effective in the world. When applied, these learned behaviors offer one an effective mix of interpersonal, strategic, and tactical experiences. To support the teachings of the Gestalt International Study Center, the following concepts and behaviors have been identified and embedded in the training, coaching, consulting and clinical work and are what differentiate Gestalt practitioners as well as those trained.

5-C Model

The "5 C-Model" is a basic tool for optimizing competence in the digital transformation. Practitioners structure competence development with different transformation models: design thinking, creativity workshops, innovation labs and more. The foundation of all these tools is the understanding of units of work and system networking. The "5-C Model" offers a common understanding of efficiency in working collaboratively. Agile working teams, scrums and other formats also find effective solutions with this model.

Level of System

Things are happening everywhere, all the time. An individual experiences anxiety, two people have an argument, a group decides to act, an organization experiences a trauma. When working with a system, we need to increase our awareness of what is happening, at what level, and determine how we want to impact the system and at what level. Do we help by talking to a senior executive in a key function or with a group of field people? Do we need to have broad communication across a group or will a personal discussion with someone make a difference? Understanding how people and organizations work allows us to see how best to influence and impact their success.

C-1: Cognition

Cognition means that the person knows the essence of what is happening in the organization and in the workplace.

The person may not know all the details but has a general overview.

Unit of Work

Each person, group or organization has any number of obligations, responsibilities, expectations, activities, tasks and other "to-dos." Each of these is at various stages of starting and completion. In Gestalt, the process of getting work done requires clarity around what it is that is being done and the stage of the cycle of experience in which we are working. Being explicit about the boundary and stage of work that is to be completed is referred to as a "unit of work." Being clear on a unit of work and completing the unit with effective closure is an important aspect of the Gestalt approach.

Multiple Realities

The Gestalt approach emphasizes the concept of multiple realities and acknowledges that we each bring our unique experience and perception to a situation and that there are always multiple ways of making meaning out of a given moment – all of which are real to the individual. We place great emphasis on teaching people how to manage differences.

C-2: Can Do

"Can do" means a person is highly professional in one or more units and is a high performer. It indicates that the person has a qualified background and/or credentials – a degree or special certificates – possesses particular business expertise or is a specialist.

C-3: Caring

Caring means that a person who knows and has the cognition of the respective organization can assume responsibilities, in case a specialist is missing, an unknown issue exists or arises in the team, or a failure emerges and needs to be resolved.

Whole-Thinking Approach

This approach is characterized by dialectical reasoning and involves understanding a system by sensing its large-scale patterns and reacting to them. Holistic thinkers believe that events are the products of external forces and situations. They tend to give broad attention to context, relationships and background elements in visual scenes.

Law of Prägnanz

This principle is also called the "law of good form." (Todorovic, 2008) Prägnanz is a German word that roughly translates as salience, incisiveness, conciseness, impressiveness, or orderliness. The understanding of Law of Prägnanz helps you to form the wholeness for your product. Making a meaningful whole for your user interface eliminates the chaotic placement of things. With using the other laws of Gestalt (similarity, proximity, continuity, closure and common fate) making a whole which is more than the sum of its parts can create a good Gestalt. This will help to create bonds between the experience you seek from users and their psychology. (Kerti, 2018)

C-4: Communicating

Communicating means that a person or group is able to communicate through constructive proposals and is able to develop and maintain a dialog with the customer and leader or with specialists inside and outside the system.

C-5: Cooperating

Cooperating means that the person or a group finds the suitable partner or a collaboration group that supports the common target achievement process.

Cooperating means furthermore that you create bonds between the thinking approaches and experiences you seek from cooperating attendees and their intents.

The 5-C Model in Practice

My team at exprobico often encounters situations in which the HR manager in a small- to medium-sized enterprise has been told, "We

need these specific performers to support our digital transformation." The list of required positions might look like this:
- Data analysts
- Data diagnostics experts
- Data translators
- Data transformers
- Data logistics managers
- Data security specialists

The HR manager then takes this information and launches a search for qualified candidates to fulfill these roles. From a Gestalt OD practitioner's perspective, management not only has not given the HR manager enough information; quite possibly, it has provided the wrong information. The practitioner might ask: Will the current workforce be considered for any of these positions? What kind of transformation is possible and meaningful with the existing staff? Has the HR manager answered these questions prior to launching a search?

Following the Whole Thinking Approach, which is characterized by dialectical reasoning and an understanding of the system's large-scale patterns, the HR manager needs a "new people business". This requires a broader understanding of human resources management than in the past. The "new people business" crosses the boundaries in a whole thinking approach before reacting to this request for new talents. HR managers, business leaders, entrepreneurs and the candidates are focusing on:
- Enabling Social Performance
- Adapting to users of new products and services
- Creating sustainability all over the world
- Understanding English language and
- Cutting Fears

Senior management can confidently say, "We have a lot of competencies." However, their HR manager must accurately assess which competencies exist and which are lacking.

What new competencies are required for a digital transformation? Is the company positioned to leverage them in the right way? How can HR managers solve this dilemma when their companies' IT managers or newly appointed Chief Digital Officers want to transform the company into a "new" world? Do the HR managers know enough about the inner workings of the tech world or do they only know the world of digital possibilities?

From a Gestalt perspective, answering these questions requires:
- Whole-Thinking Approach
- Cross-Boundary Networking
- Collaboration and Communication
- Interdisciplinary Teamwork
- Decision Making on the Spot

This calls for collaborative work. The "5-C Model" can facilitate and support that.

The System-Thinking Approach

Let's follow a first Gestalt principle, the "Level of Systems." In traditional organizations, we usually have an organizational structure with a very strong hierarchical format. No one has documented the "real" operational structure. On paper, an org chart supposedly illustrates how the enterprise operates; but it is not the reality. Numerous systems function simultaneously and/or interactively within that organization.

If we follow the value chain, we can detect very different systems involving customers and suppliers inside and outside the organization, logistics, delivery, warehousing, quality assurance, etc. We observe single-person systems, groups, teams, leaders, collaborative partners and customer systems.

Let's examine the different levels of systems from the perspective of a new team leader in the assembly department of a mechanical engineering company: He started his career there as a fitter. He wanted to do a great job, but quickly realized that he could not succeed if he did not cooperate with the electrician in the early phases of assembly. In other words, he knew he needed to interact well with another system to be successful. But that wasn't all.

As he progressed in the role, he became more familiar with all the other systems in his organization. He kept himself fully informed about any news or changes in the business, communicated with others as they expected, and designed processes to make his job as efficient as possible. That worked very well for years.

This fitter thrived because he kept the big picture in mind. He was productive and proficient, understood how his company functioned and he knew how to maximize his effectiveness within it. He personified the C-1 (cognition) and C-2 (can do) elements of the 5-C Model.

As time progressed, his company increased their product mix and the throughput of its machines. At the same time, they shortened their lead times. Logistics, materials provisioning, deadlines, purchased parts, quality assurance, as well as acceptance audits from customers changed the requirements placed on the company's assembly activity. It also changed the cooperation the fitter needed to deliver the required outcomes: high-quality, customer-specific machines. It meant that he could no longer focus solely on the cooperation of the internal assembly team.

The company needed someone to coordinate all of these functions but could not afford to hire someone to function solely as a manager. Consequently, the fitter and team leader roles were combined, and the high-performing fitter was considered for a promotion. The combined roles would create a high stress level for him and everyone around him. Did this high-performing fitter have the potential to advance?

Our competency check revealed that this fitter had developed and nurtured the necessary relationships inside and outside of the company. He also had the best cognition of the systems involved in the assembly environment. We then coached him on leveraging his potential as a team leader.

The Unit of Work

The second Gestalt principle, "Unit of Work," supported our understanding of the core competencies of each member of this team – fitters, electricians and other functions (systems) within the organization – and the responsibilities of the team leaders and others. To bring transparency in complex systems, our task is to determine what the units of work are; what the input is; what the beginning, middle and especially the end points are; and what the outcome of the unit is.

Because there were other areas of the company undergoing transformation, there were numerous units of work to complete before the company accomplished its transformation goals. We conducted numerous workshops with all the stakeholders to determine what the individual units were. As a result, we were able to clarify the roles and the process itself. As we visualized all findings on flipcharts and built landscapes on the floor, we found ourselves struggling with boundaries and responsibilities.

We trained more people in the organization, as we had done with the fitter. Together with a senior manager, we eventually developed a group of team leaders who possessed C-1 (cognition) and C-2 (can do) in a broader range of level of systems and within different roles. This provided each with insights into leadership.

The company had not labeled this process as digitalization and transformation, but it was. They were transforming their old paper-based environment into a digitally supported world. For the new team leaders throughout the various systems of the organization, using business tools such as SAP, quality reports, IT support, order systems and programming new machines was an enormous challenge.

The transformation required a new vocabulary. There were English-speaking customers who communicated via e-mail. The current and future complexity of information, networking, products and services were explained using unfamiliar names. No one seemed to understand each other.

Frustrated, some of the "older" leaders changed positions. Young newcomers jumped into the cold water and realized quickly that they needed to upgrade their skills and knowledge base. They quit.

We noticed a considerable lack of responsibility. Wherever we checked, one question dominated: "Who cares?"

Multiple Realities

The third C, Caring, is strongly related to the Gestalt principle of Multiple Realities within a system and organizations.

We have worked with manufacturing organizations. Some described the devices they produce in terms of their value to the marketplace and the benefits they deliver. It should be noted that these were the company's intended benefits, seen solely from the company's reality. There could be other realities. Perhaps this device could function differently, or its features and benefits could be perceived differently.

There are multiple realities within the larger system, as well. Senior management's reality could differ from their middle managers' or their customers'. Each reality is reflected in their priorities and choices.

To purchasing managers, cost is a priority, so they might buy large volumes to receive a bulk discount. Logistics managers also want to save money, but their reality is that it would be wasteful to buy 1,000 widgets when they only need 10.

Meanwhile, the company's quality manager is laser-focused on each device meeting 100% of the quality standards. The operations manager also wants to deliver the highest quality products but has a larger reality: assuring that all departments function like a well-oiled machine because the general sales manager needs a shorter throughput. The sales department has acquired new customers, and that manager now has to meet those customers' reality.

During workshops with these managers, we discussed the different realities and engaged them in Units of Work exercises. The feedback was positive. After completing the exercises, they reported a more solid grasp of the meaning of boundaries. The workshops also enabled them to connect with each other in the same room, which deepened their understanding of how the work of others contributed to their own set of tasks.

This level of interdepartmental communication had not previously occurred. Over time, some leaders had lost their voice. Instead of speaking directly with their counterparts to address a problem, they communicated electronically, had a lot of clashes and blamed the computer systems.

Were they doing something wrong? No. It was merely a lack of communication in the first place and a lack of understanding of multiple realities in the second place.

To help them develop competence in this area, we took a Gestalt approach. We worked with single groups of the system and with individuals. We pictured in a positive way what the realities of the others were and discussed how that reality benefited the entire system. Then we asked them to "jump into the moccasins of the others" so they could develop their own action plan – but from their counterpart's viewpoint.

We have found communications to be an excellent tool for clarifying multiple realities. Individuals can reduce complexity overall by communicating the facts and dialoging about these issues. It generates understanding and transparency. Even if the issues are very complex, it does not mean the communication about them must be complicated.

To resolve an issue, everyone simply needs to know the end goal and how their actions will affect the achievement of that goal. They need to answer questions such as:
- Who can take care of the case if something does not fit?
- How do we take care of it?

- With whom do we communicate?
- How do we cooperate with each other?

In the case of the mechanical engineering company, what the team leaders discovered through this process was that the pure assembly process – something they considered a core competence and core process – was actually a "secondary competence" in the digital transformation. The top-level competence was the disposition and coordination, cooperation and control of the appropriate IT systems. That competence determined the efficiency of the assembly.

Once they discovered this, they were able to see that the role of the fitter was more pivotal to the success of the whole than they had previously envisioned. Consequently, it was assigned managerial status – even if the same person was performing the task and managing the department.

As the new fitter/team leader became more and more involved with his partners in the process, he became a more valuable service provider for his assembly colleagues as each of them learned and mastered the secondary competence: the new IT systems.

Leveraging the Gestalt approach during this transformation process also revealed that all core competencies in assembly process had to be further improved, from the ergonomics of the assembly processes to the interaction of operating resources such as workstations, tools and fixtures. This required conceptual work and design know-how – fields of competence that had not previously been considered.

Prior to our involvement, assembly employees acted independently, and assembly departments worked in silos. Directions came from the top and decisions were made without collaboration. Incorporating the C-5 Model enabled them to redesign the workplace with input from the assembly workers. That input was then communicated to the specialty departments, which accomplished another transformation competence.

The Whole-Thinking Approach

Today, the new fitter/team leader's role has evolved and expanded to include cooperative learning processes across departments. There is now an exchange of knowledge, communication and coordination with those who work within his assembly area and in the service and control areas. His goal aligns with the company's newly desired competency: A workplace in which everyone is engaged in a learning process that improves the proficiency of their core tasks, and they understand how their performance of those tasks impacts the business's success.

By embracing a more Gestalt approach, the company was able to surpass its initial goal of introducing new technology. Instead, it inspired the workforce to operate and cooperate effectively and efficiently with that new technology.

The team leaders and the whole system regularly applied the "5-C Model," from C-1 to C-5: whenever the environment changed, system boundaries had to be crossed, or when a basic competence became obsolete. Robots may one day perform the fitter's role, but the foundational competence of knowing the desired unit of work and networking with others is not as easily replaced.

The whole-thinking approach also enabled team leaders and teams to develop new competencies, including difficult high-level social skills:
- Dealing with criticism and mistakes
- Rethinking, coming out of old behavior patterns
- Overcoming the fear of something new
- Understanding new job requirements – technological and other processes – and fields of action

This approach further enhanced team leaders' value to their company. They became viewed as specialists. They were trusted to determine which actions to take and which hardware and software best supported the digital transformation.

They also contributed valuable insights for improving employee efficiency because they had gained competence in determining the units of work and how to optimize them. If they continue to work with the 5-C Model, they will always one step ahead of the transformation process.

The success of transformations such as this prompted confirms the efficacy of the exprobico competence check and affirms the sage advice of experts such as Peter F. Drucker (2001), who stated, "If you can't measure it, you can't improve it." I should add that measuring competencies also enables boundaries to be visible and helps individuals and teams develop sound solutions.

Our relationships and interactions are becoming more global, and individuals are becoming more flexible and future-oriented, which requires us to be lifelong learners. And that can be exciting. As Fritz Perls[6] once said, "To learn means to discover something is possible."

My team is now better equipped to determine team members' and leaders' core competencies and assess how they align with digital transformation requirements. In addition, by following and applying the 5 C Model, we can ease them into this new world without raising fear anxiety.

Moreover, using this model facilitates a better understanding of change, whether a company is shifting from a paper-based environment to a digital one, incorporating younger tech-savvy employees into an established older workforce or trying to overcome language barriers created by the merger or acquisition of a foreign company. After all, even the tech world has its own language.

Conclusion

Interacting with Gestalt-based methods, processes and tools enables us to master complexity in a simple, comprehensible way. We need boundaries in order to change and develop. Therefore, we also need holistic approaches and tools, measuring instruments and procedures that make us aware of these boundaries so we can transcend them consciously and efficiently and leverage our potentials holistically.

References

Drucker, Peter (2000). *The Essential Drucker.* Abingdon, UK: Taylor & Francis Ltd.

ExploringYourMind.com (2018). *The Best Fritz Perls Quotes* [online], available at https://exploringyourmind.com/the-35-best-fritz-perls-quotes/

Kerti, Erkan (2018). *The Designer's Guide to the Law of Prägnanz, Fundamental principle of the Gestalt Theory,* [online], available at https://blog.prototypr.io/law-of-prägnanz-bdb2fcf349b8

Todorovic, D. (2008). Gestalt Principles, *Scholarpedia.* [online], available at http://www.scholarpedia.org/article/Gestalt_principles

Chapter 15: Leading Change: A Gestalt Perspective

Jonno Hanafin

"Stability doesn't exist. The world changes with every breath"

Buddhist saying

Gestalt theories, models and principles provide a powerful and practical set of lenses through which the challenges of leading change can be examined and exploited. The holistic aspect of Gestalt ensures leaders and interveners consider the context, consequences and complexity of any system they influence. The Gestalt notion of boundaries as the relationship between organism and environment (O/E,) provides a meaningful framework for organizing thinking about leading and managing change.

Leading versus managing is a false dichotomy when it comes to leading change. Managing is about working within established boundaries. Leading is about rearranging the boundaries. They overlap: managers do lead (within boundaries), and leaders do manage (across boundaries). In leading change, there is as much to manage as there is to lead. The key lies in what the change leader is managing.

Managers are responsible for executing the strategy, implementing the business plan and operating the day-to-day enterprise. Managers solve problems. A problem is a situation requiring attention and correction, whether it's an empty fuel tank or a dysfunctional organization process. There is a solution to the problem. Leaders manage dilemmas (Hanafin, 1998). A dilemma is the existence of inherently conflicting forces at work in a system (e.g., focusing on short-term results or long-term results, doing what's best for the customer or what's best for the company). Dilemmas cannot be solved; they can only be managed. All relationships are dilemmas, including the relationship between organism and environment. There is no way to eliminate the tension from a dilemma. It just has to be managed as well as possible under the circumstances.

CEOs exclusively manage dilemmas as they carry out their three primary responsibilities: strategy, culture and succession. Strategy is board-approved. Culture includes values. Succession includes the procurement and development of talent. Many CEOs see talent as the single most important success variable. Leaders at all levels wear multiple hats: inspiration provider, visionary, strategist, planner, role model, talent developer and change agent. In many ways, leadership itself is a dilemma: constantly juggling and rebalancing the competing forces from a variety of stakeholders.

Disruption is both a driver and a consequence of change. It can be internally propelled (e.g., reorganizing or acquiring,) or externally forced (e.g., a new competitor in the market or breakthrough technology.) Change is relentless, ruthless and can be lightning fast. Some battery technology, for example, is obsolete before it reaches the market. Whether preemptive or reactive, the leader is accountable for guiding the introduction and implementation of the change. Staying abreast of the ever-changing environment demands change leaders be chronic learners.

Unit of Work

The skill set required to lead change successfully is primarily learned from experience (own and others), over time. While we learn most effectively from experience, having experience is no guarantee we learn from it. The difference between having experience and learning from it can be found in the Unit of Work model (Carter, 2004), a simple and powerful framework for thinking about processes of any complexity. Consider any unit of work (a project, a meeting, an assignment) as having three phases: a beginning, a middle and an end. This framework is grounded in our cultures in the form of fairy tales: "Once upon a time", story, "they lived happily ever after." The principal difference between having experience and learning from it is attending to the end of a unit of work where learning takes place. It is largely a matter of asking, "What did we learn from what we just experienced?"

UNIT OF WORK

Beginning	Middle	End
"Once Upon a Time"	Story	"They Lived Happily Ever After"
Phase I	Phase II	Phase III
Launch	Direct/Manage	Sustain
Context	Contact	Closure
Clarify intent & path	Execute	Close & learn

The classic change model (Lewin, 1951) ("unfreeze–change–refreeze") deserves to be revisited. The notion of a period of stability between changes no longer holds true in many arenas. Most leaders recognize the need for changing on the fly. Many, in fast paced organizations, complain of having "no time to think." This is true, even in the case of organizations that advertise themselves as thought leaders.

The Performance–Learning Dilemma

Which is more important in any role: that we perform or that we learn? The answer is 'yes.' When the answer to a multiple choice question is 'all of the above,' this is a dilemma. The performance–learning dilemma in many organizations is lopsided in favor of performance. Because results matter so much, the learning side of the polarity is undervalued. Hence, many leaders and organizations repeatedly make the same mistakes. (Consider politicians who fail to realize that the cover-up is worse than the crime.) When a project is completed, there is a strong tendency to move on to the next challenge, often exacerbated by the formidable plate of work remaining. Taking time to extract learning from what was just completed seems like a luxury (with the exception of blame expeditions in pursuit of finding fault.) Hard-earned learning is often left on the table.

Regardless of a company's business advantage, the only true sustainable competitive advantage is to learn faster than the competition. Whatever competitive edge an organization has, it can eventually be done faster, cheaper or reverse engineered by someone else. Passing over a learning debrief in the interest of saving time is like touring European castles and not getting off the bus. When individuals, groups, organizations and larger social systems deprive themselves of a chance to learn from their experience, they forego fresh insight. "No time to think" becomes "no time to learn;" hardly a mantra for competitive advantage. The Gestalt model advocates for the whole experience, including the ending. Healthy interaction with the environment results in change, learning and growth.

The Phases of Leading Change

As noted in the Unit of Work model, every change project can be viewed through the lens of a beginning, middle and end, or Phases I – III. Phase I is about setting the context, launching, initiating and developing traction. Phase II is about managing and directing the change process to ensure contact is made. Phase III is about sustaining the change, closure and learning.

Phase I – Launching the Change: Announcement is Not a Change Strategy

The leader provides the rationale for initiating change and will execute one of two fundamental change models. One is the vision model, based on a compelling aspirational picture of a future state (e.g., healthcare for everyone, product within arm's reach of everyone on the planet). It is based on the leader's vision and the quantum physics principle that energy follows thought: i.e., 'we move toward the pictures we create.' (Carter, 1993.) The attractiveness of the vision draws organization members' energy and commitment. The only thing more powerful than a compelling vision is a shared vision. Leadership teams need to report more on their process and shared passion, in addition to the vision statement they unveil.

The other change model is the awareness model, based on the Paradoxical Theory of Change (Beisser, 1970). The Paradoxical Theory states that change happens when we become more of who we are, not when we try to be different. The development task is to heighten awareness of what is, the fundamental Gestalt growth strategy. The starting place is collecting data on the current state; conducting an employee engagement survey, for example. Analysis of the data will result in themes that suggest areas requiring attention. The urge to improve provides the impetus for initiating change. For example, in individual performance reviews, growth happens when one is given challenging feedback about the impact of one's behavior. The individual then chooses to modify her behavior or not. Providing feedback that someone needs to be different typically serves to heighten resistance.

Whether the vision model or the awareness model is used, leaders have to pay attention to how the change is introduced. There are a number of pitfalls inherent in the presentation. Among them, the belief that an announcement is a change strategy. It is not. Unveiling the desired change doesn't change anything except the anxiety level in the organization due to the level of uncertainty that has been introduced.

Consider the rising stress level that follows the online posting of a new org chart. The first thing people ask when a change of any kind is announced is, "What about me?" The sexiest new vision, the smartest new strategy and the long-anticipated acquisition take second place to self-concern. After the announcement, leaders must manage the impact on individuals. Meet with people and openly share as much as is known. It is better to have a conversation and admit that all the impact of the change is not yet known than to remain silent.

One Canadian CEO, in the midst of searching for a new partner to save a joint venture, met with all employees every Friday afternoon during the course of the search. Even if there was nothing new to report, convening people for discussion, support and rumor-sharing provided a degree of comfort that helped mitigate the anxiety inherent in the "will-we-or-won't-we-survive" situation. Well-intended leaders often assume they should wait until they have all the information. In the absence of information, people make up their own movies (projection), and the movies they make up are usually much worse than what is being considered.

No matter how appealing the change may appear, there is an implicit criticism in any change: The way we were doing it was wrong. Although it won't necessarily be spoken or even felt initially, people need to hear that the way they have been doing things up until now was right. This is a manifestation of the systems principle that all systems are functioning as best they can at any moment. Things have changed and now we have the opportunity to do better. Making the statement explicit preempts unconscious defensiveness later.

Millennials, more than other generational groups, need the case for change to make sense. They are not moved by authority, reward or conformance. Leaders need to create a different narrative tailored to each member constituency group.

Phase II – Directing the Change: Managing Dilemmas

The leading-change skill set includes a variety of elements for the change leader to manage in executing a change process. These include a number of Gestalt-based perspectives, strategies and dilemmas.

Congruence and Credibility: The Words and the Music

Once the intent (the why and what) of the change initiative is communicated, attention shifts to the how of implementing. Tracking the degree of alignment is crucial for credibility. Putting out a vision statement is a courageous act, because once it is made public, people immediately focus on the gap between where the organization aspires to be and where it actually is. This gap can be experienced as leadership hypocrisy. Leaders can minimize this sentiment by acknowledging upfront the long journey to realizing the desired state. Providing the general strategy and path toward the vision also helps address the skepticism.

The strongest determinant of leadership credibility during a change is the alignment between the rhetoric and the perceived reality: what leaders say and what they do. When the words and the music don't match, people follow the music. Leaders can say what they want, but organization members take their cues from watching how leaders conduct themselves. Nothing is more powerful in promoting or dismissing the relevance of the values than leader behavior, especially in times of stress. One public high school system in Colorado, committed to a values-based culture, assembles students and teachers each morning before class to share examples of behavior consistent with the stated values. Those whose behavior deviated from the values are given the opportunity to speak publicly about their transgression and learning. This includes faculty. The school system has the highest performance rating in the state and 100% college acceptances.

Change Strategies: Four More

The vision- and awareness-heightening strategies noted earlier serve to pull and push organizations in new directions. There are additional strategies available to the change leader, including role modeling, restructuring, reward system and education.

Role Modeling – Arguably the most powerful and undervalued change strategy. People mimic the behavior of those in leadership positions, consciously when they respect them and unconsciously when they don't. Everything a leader says or does, doesn't say or do is a message to the organization. People read between the lines to gauge how they are expected to conduct themselves. This is especially true in the case of a new leader when organization members vie to learn quickly what approaches and behavior will now be rewarded. These leader messages are often unintentional, but they are powerful nonetheless. Effective change leaders are intentional in displaying how they want their followers to behave. One of the quickest ways new CEOs begin shaping the culture they inherit is their own language, meeting behavior, dress and questions they ask. For those whose response to a call for new behavior is wait-and-see, modeling gives them something to see. Leaders are always teaching.

Restructuring – Probably the most preferred and least powerful change strategy. Its attractiveness is its apparent simplicity. Redraw the boxes and lines. Rearranging boundaries and reporting relationships usually provides more a shift that is more optical than substantive; but it does send a signal. The structural approach creates visible change quickly; but it must be supplemented with strong engagement follow-up that clarifies new roles and relationships, aligns expectations, contracts power and authority). Structure does impact behavior over time. For example, in matrixed organizations, the primary determinant of loyalty is geographic proximity. Structure change may be necessary, but it is usually not sufficient.

Reward System – People do what they get rewarded for. Reward refers to recognition, as well as financial. Acknowledgement is a powerful force. When it comes to promoting fresh ways of thinking and new behavior, catching someone doing it right and drawing attention to it is a reinforcement opportunity. The leader is teaching, using someone else's behavior.

Education – A traditionally popular change strategy, requiring updating. If people are expected to develop different ways of thinking and behaving, they need exposure to other ways of operating. New behavior requires new skills. Mindset is one of those skills – a possibility or growth mindset, for example. Short-term behavior change can be forced by fear and intimidation, but sustainable behavior change must be connected to new ways of thinking. As illustrated below, enduring behavior change requires going further upstream in the process.

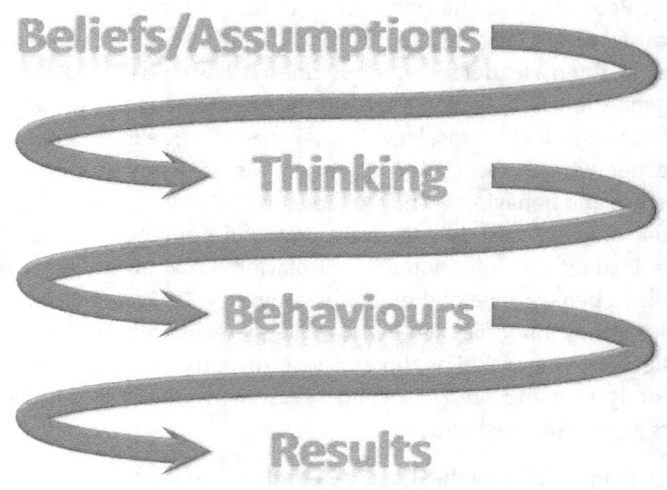

Expressed differently:

> If I continue to believe what I have always believed,
> I will continue to think as I have always thought.
>
> If I continue to think as I have always thought,
> I will continue to act as I have always acted.
>
> If I continue to act as I have always acted,
> I will continue to get what I have always gotten.

This is an extended version of the vernacular definition of insanity, i.e. doing the same thing and expecting a different outcome. The deeper the shift (i.e., beliefs and assumptions), the more embedded the change will be.

Traditional acquisitional learning through lectures, videos, slide decks and testimonials is not as powerful as experiential learning. Designing experiential learning is a distinctive art and science. It relies more on development than training, focuses more on outcome intent than script, and relies more on in-the-moment facilitators than trainers or presenters. The Gestalt methodology of co-creating and facilitating experiments greatly enhances this skill set.

Given the Paradoxical Theory of Change, the development task with any education model is supporting people to be more of who they are, not different than who they are. This translates to helping people expand their range and is done by provoking people in a supportive and challenging way to the edge of their comfort zone, or contact boundary. At any level of organization change, growth and comfort do not co-exist.

Managing the Dilemma of Resistance: Harness the Energy

Any force for change is met with a force for maintaining the status quo (Lewin, 1951). Ambivalence is the natural state. Human beings and organizations are not binary, but more like a dimmer switch. Even if the leader wants to initiate change, there is a part of him, however small, that prefers leaving things as they are. It's less work; the familiar is more comfortable. Likewise, even if members don't want to change, part of them does; it's exciting, and there are things about the status quo they don't like.

For status quo, we can use the language of persistence, or as is more often the case, resistance. Resistance has a negative connotation, as in something to be overcome or destroyed. The change leader's first step in dealing with resistance is to reframe it. Gestalt theory views resistance as an inevitable and healthy force. It is energy in a different direction. That energy needs to be captured, not eliminated. Resistance is the activation of an organism's immune system, the self-preservation urge of cultures. It serves to regulate change. Unless cultures are architected to welcome difference, they perceive threat. For example, many companies acquired as part of a roll-up strategy resist centralizing customer care. This can be seen as resistance to being controlled by new ownership. Experienced acquisition leaders appreciate this persistence as a commitment to staying close to their loyal customers.

One successful CEO recognized that "the more you push them, the more they resist." His approach was seductive and Socratic: let the acquired entities lead themselves to the change. He acknowledged their valid concerns, told them they could decide, then shared all the metrics and best practice information with them. Their defensiveness morphed into curiosity and they eventually adopted the change, as they saw it was best for their business. He didn't take the bait of false efficiency (it's faster to just command it). His view was that it took a little longer than he would have preferred, but the overall time to change was actually shorter since it would have taken longer dealing with resistance (recycle.) He allowed the acquired companies to control the pace of transition.

The strategy for dealing with resistance is to respect it, go with it and channel it in the interest of shared goals. Resistance is a source of energy. It is easier to harness energy than to create it. The effective change leader responds to resistance with curiosity – "Isn't that interesting?" (Nevis, 1987) – rather than defensiveness.

Managing Experiments: Converting to Action

One of the challenges in leading change is translating lofty visions and goals into action. This is done using experiments. Experiments are a way of enlivening and generating energy in an organization. Models don't change anything. Experiments convert those ideas into action, experience and insight. Experiments are about trying something and learning. They are based on identified themes, such as improving innovation or ramping up collaboration. High-control organizations shy away from using experiments because the outcome is not known in advance. Experiments must be designed in a way that creates what Gestalt calls a "safe emergency." The amount of safety and risk must be calibrated. Too much of either will not result in learning or change. An experiment can be as simple as allocating five minutes at the end of every meeting to debrief, or as complex as setting up a parallel skunkworks organization. Both mobilize energy and have the objective of learning how to improve performance.

Experiments and rituals occupy opposite ends of the continuum, and both have their place as tools for the change leader. Rituals support stability and building culture. Experiments support change and improvement.

Managing Boundaries: Where Change Takes Place

Where is the line between the real world and the virtual world? What is the right mix of preservers and innovators? In some organizations what used to be required is no longer needed. These are boundary management issues. The Gestalt concept of Organism/Environment (O/E) noted above provides a useful frame for exploring the relationship between any entity and its context. Boundaries can lose their flexibility and permeability over time. Overly rigid organizations become bureaucracies at the expense of innovation. People are rewarded for compliance, not creation. Change leaders create a work environment that encourages constant monitoring and modifying established norms, processes and structures in the service of improvement.

Imagine a seven-year-old looking at the stars and seeing a spaceship. Telling her no, it is Sagittarius, is like saying, "That's the way we've always done it" in an over- bounded organization.

Boundaries provide definition for things such as roles: how the organization relates to its environment, what people are rewarded for. They give meaning by setting limits. Without limitations we can be left floating in a sea of possibilities. Leaders provide the definition (strategy, values, culture) within which managers can execute. They also challenge the underlying assumptions (often inherited) for relevance in the current situation and teach others to do the same. Perhaps the most useful boundary a change leader provides is clarity about what is **not** changing, such as the company's values. Defining the baby so it can be distinguished from the bathwater prevents unnecessary resistance and promotes focus.

Managing Self: Maintaining the Equipment

The greatest tool the change leader possesses is herself. Leaders are catalysts. In chemistry, some catalysts are consumed in the process. This is not the desired model. The first rule of thumb for change agents is Stay Alive (Shepard, 1975). While self-sacrifice in the cause of change may be noble, it is not practical. Change leaders need to ensure they are maintaining the equipment to be their best self. Self preventive maintenance, built on a holistic platform of physical, spiritual and emotional wellbeing includes reliable direct feedback, regular stimulation, reflection opportunities and a strong support system. Self-care is not a selfish act. Consider the Buddhist saying: "One cannot pour from an empty cup."

Nearly every leadership framework currently offered contains a high level of self-awareness in its model. Self-awareness is a prerequisite for use of self with intentionality and informed choice. It also supports a presence of openness, which is necessary for true engagement; i.e., the Gestalt notion of 'contact' with mutual influence. One Latin American general manager participated in a two-day workshop designed for his senior lead. When asked at the end why he took the time away from his busy job to join them, he said, "You can't expect people to trust you if they don't know you."

Phase III – Learning, Closure and Sustainability: The Harvest

Endings are generally not the most popular stage in processes. There is more excitement at beginnings and more intensity in the middle. When the end comes, people are often eager to move on to what's next. But shortcutting the ending is like planting and tending to crops – then walking away before the harvest.

Learning takes place at the end. Taking time to ask, "What did we learn from what we just experienced?" is how individuals, teams and organizations create wisdom and preempt repetition of mistakes. Organizations committed to capturing competitive advantage are fanatical about this learning stage.

Closure means finishing what can be finished and acknowledging what cannot. Unfinished business keeps coming around until it is finished. One international resource company merged all its regional headquarters into one global headquarters, reducing headcount by 50%. There was no processing of the change, and no curiosity about retention criteria and survivor guilt. Three years later, during the data collection phase for a diversity initiative, the number-one grievance in interviews was the headquarters consolidation. Unfinished business wastes energy and detracts focus. Closure builds the trust level in organizations.

Often the change morphs into a different form, perhaps the beginning of another change effort. The ending is the opportunity to build in sustainability. What mechanisms will ensure the momentum continues? How can the learning be fed forward to a new group or initiative? The change leader is as responsible for a robust conclusion as a strong start.

Conclusion

Growth doesn't come without change, and change doesn't come without discomfort. Leaders are change agents. They manage the discomfort of a dynamic process by providing guidance, clarity and a visible model of how to navigate the uncertainty together. Leaders versed in a Gestalt stance derive confidence in dealing with the 'what is' of any situation.

References

Hanafin, J. (1998). Problems and Dilemmas. *Gestalt Institute of Cleveland International Organization and Systems Development Program Course Material,* The Netherlands: Gestalt Institute of Cleveland.

Carter, J. (2004). Carter's Cube and a Gestalt/OSD Toolbox: A Square, a Circle, a Triangle and a Line. *OD Practitioner,* 36(4), pp. 11-17.

Lewin, K. (1951). *Field theory in social science.* New York: Harper.

Beisser, A. (1970). The aradoxical theory of change. In: J. Fagan, J. & I. Shepherd, I. ed., *Gestalt Therapy Now: Theory, Techniques, Applications.* Palo Alto: Gestalt Journal Press.

Nevis, E. (1987). Organizational consulting: A Gestalt approach. Cambridge, MA: Gestalt Press.

Shepard, H. (1985). Rules of thumb for change agents. In: D. Kolb, I. Rubin and J. Osland, ed. *The organizational behavior reader, 5th ed.* Englewood Cliffs, NJ: Prentice Hall, pp. 682-689.

Carter, J., Hirsch, L., Kepner, E., Lukensmeyer, C. and Nevis, E. (1977). *Gestalt Institute of Cleveland Organization and Systems Development Program Course Material.* Cleveland: Gestalt Institute of Cleveland.

Rainey Tolbert, M.A. and Hanafin, J. (2006). Use of Self in OD Consulting: What Matters is Presence. In: *The NTL Handbook of Organization Development and Change.* San Francisco: Pfeiffer, pp. 69-82.

Rainey, M.A. and Stratford, C. (2001) Reframing resistance to change: A Gestalt perspective. In: G. Bermann and G. Meurer, ed. *Best Patterns – Erfolgsmuster für zukunftsfähiges Management.* Berlin: Hermann Luchterhand Verlag, GmbH, Neuwied und Kriftel, pp. 327-336.

Von Bertalanffy, L. (1988). *General system theory: Foundations, development, and applications,* Revised ed. New York: Braziller.

Cotham, F. (2006) 'I hope this isn't meant to be a criticism' [Cartoon]. *New Yorker,* 12 June.

Chapter 16: A Systemic Gestalt Supporting Transformational Change: Using the Six C's

Brenda B. Jones

The 21st century is a time of unprecedented and unpredictable change. To address change and thrive in this environment requires multiple perspectives, new frameworks, and the courage to take risks and be innovative. The constant disruption, uncertainty and ambiguity fuels feelings that life and the world, in general, are unimaginably complicated and the challenges are insurmountable. Additionally, three paradoxes that organizations historically face make managing change even more complex: Organizations don't change unless they have to. Second, organizations find it increasingly difficult, even when motivated, to make changes to adjust to trends, develop talent and meet growth targets. Finally, it's difficult for organizations to stop looking back to past successes, move on to commit to changes that are mostly uncomfortable, and venture into the unknown.

In his book, *The Age of The Unthinkable*, Joshua Cooper Ramo (2010) states that successful organizations develop resilience, which he defines as the ability to learn and get stronger from each unexpected challenge instead of crumbling under the pressure of a rapidly changing environment. Organizations must foster an environment conducive to changing dynamics by accelerating learning, challenging assumptions and experimenting more in order to take bolder actions.

A Gestalt and Systems Approach to Change

Gestalt practices speak to these contemporary tensions now, possibly more than they did in the 20th century. Gestalt theory, concepts and models are a powerful orientation for growth and change as they address the experience of the individual, the group and the organization at the core of the work. In life and in organizations, it is important to discover unique ways of understanding self/individual and making meaning.

As a Gestalt practitioner, O (Organism)/E (Environment), Figure/Ground, and Field Theory are three central Gestalt Theory and Concepts. They are described as follows:

1. O (Organism)/E (Environment) Organizations is the organism with a boundary in and of itself. It is not isolated from the environment, but has an ongoing relationship with others for the phenomenological learning of the organization. Yontef (1993)
2. Figure/Ground: A figure is an image, object or subject on which a person focuses his or her attention. The ground is the background or environment that is within the person's awareness.
3. Field Theory: The organism's experience is explored in the context of its situation or environment. Lewin (1936) wrote about the importance of the atmosphere and the amount of freedom existing in the situation.

Systems theory and thinking are ways to understand the interconnectedness of the parts and to provide an understanding of the whole. Having a systems perspective with respect to change means recognizing all parts of the organization. Systems thinking also refers to different levels of system – individuals, groups and the organization – which are interacting with and affecting each other simultaneously. (Jones 2014)

As such, the effect of Gestalt and Systems Theories can help heighten one's awareness, develop an open system view and value experimentation as keys to approaching change and transformation. These perspectives can be integrative with a w/holistic view of the organization and its environment. The interest in the whole system being healthy can bring new understandings to growth and change, shifting mindsets and behaviors and, thereby, producing results.

Building Blocks of a New Gestalt Perspective

Throughout this chapter the process of change is examined from both Gestalt and System perspectives in organizations. These perspectives become the foundation for the development of the 3 C's plus 3 C's approach. The primacy of all of the C's provides a dynamic view of the two sets of C's creating a strong and useful "Gestalt" about change and transformation.

The first set of 3 C's (context, consciousness and culture) builds strong figures that give levels of understanding to complex change and transformation efforts. Each C supports the adaptive challenges described by Heifetz (2002) in his familiar metaphor of how perspectives and actions vary when viewed from the "dance floor" or from a "balcony" overlooking the dance floor. Each view is filtered through a strategic, complex and catalyst lens. This set of C's take a balcony and systems view. The intention of this zooming out process gives an internal and external picture and perspective of critical parts of an organizational change and transformation. Decisions from this process can drive direction and results. Individually and together these C's can create energy, momentum and unexpected opportunities for alignment. They provide the bounding and grounding efforts for a stronger position for the organization to bring clarity.

The second set of 3 C's (capacity, capability and competency) represent the development of the individual, group and the organization. While each C can be viewed as a separate entity, to successfully address profound challenges requires holding all of C's in consideration. It is the definition of each C and the integration in the meaning making that brings relevance and importance to a real sense about learning and change. This intelligence can provide deeper and expansive growth opportunities, new ways to learn, develop and mature at the individual, group and organization level of system.

Adult Learning and Development

A critical key to change and transformation is to cultivate a learning stance as much as a performance stance. Adult ego development theory distinguishes growth stages in emotional, cognitive, physical and spiritual levels and develops the ability to move beyond subjective thinking to become more objective. The development process must include growth in both vertical and horizontal directions Petrie (2014). Horizontal development is acquiring subject specific knowledge and competencies that deepen perceptions and task performance. Vertical development is the acquiring of mental complexity, allowing emotional and relational capacities to increase. Vertical development is characterized by intense stretch experiences (the what), new ways of thinking (the how) and strong developmental networks (the who). Ultimately, this development improves how one interprets the world, strategically and systemically thinks, and manages conflict (Brown, 2012). Individuals and organizations will need to learn as rapidly with changes occurring in the environment in order to experience successful transformation(s).

Out of the Field and the Ground

Kurt Lewin's (1936) aim is to represent the field 'correctly, as it exists for the individual in question at a particular time.' Field Theory is inextricably linked to this exploration of change and transformation across levels of systems. It becomes important to understand, explain, predict or change human behavior while taking into account the organism in relation to its environment.

Taking a broad view of the field, an organization is able to get a wide-ranging perspective to meet the challenge or use opportunity to face its goals. The field refers to: (a) all aspects of individuals in relationship with their surroundings and conditions; (b) that apparently influence the particular behaviors and developments of concern; (c) at a particular point in time. When paying attention to the field, multiple figures emerge that give shape to the big picture and create an objective condition within which the organization perceives and acts.

In an age of exponential change, the actions of an organization must be informed by stakeholders' perspective from an outside in view as much as an inside out view. This enables people in organizations to take more risks, identify options and make better choices from a broad field. As a Gestalt practitioner, the process can help organizations mature and identify critical figures on which they can focus their attention to characterize the change and ensure deliberate action. Heightening awareness and making choices supports an organization's responses to the current realities. A culture of constant learning and self-evaluation allows organizations to survive and thrive in a competitive environment.

Understanding Context, Consciousness and Culture

The effectiveness of action depends upon the clarity and understanding of context, consciousness and culture of the most robust figures in the field. This will identify sources that spring from the richness in the ground and possibly allow recognition of new opportunities to shift towards during the coming years. It is imperative to have a sense of organization in relation to the field. Otherwise, the field itself can leave a system too under-bounded or too over-bounded. Andrew McAfee

(2013) would call this time of change and transformation "the second half of the chessboard" saying we haven't seen anything yet. The first set of C's can help to develop a clear and compelling view of the landscape.

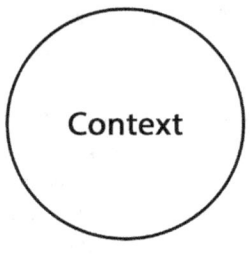

Everything operates in a context. Context is the circumstances or facts that surround and impact a particular system, event, situation, etc. By not being aware of what is happening, an individual or organization loses the ability to respond appropriately, prepare for disruption or position for the future. Context answers the questions, "What am I/we aware of right now?" and "What are the internal and external factors and conditions we must be aware of?"

Context provides perspective and some preverbal "dots" even when they cannot yet be connected. This is the understanding of the "what is" and "what if" that gives insights about the present as well as about the potential future. It is important to observe and stay curious about unknown conditions that could affect the current situation.

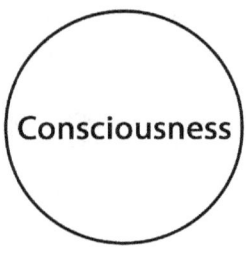

Consciousness is grounded in phenomenology and is ambiguous and complex. Something happens and nothing happens and both create consciousness. It is part of the understanding, complexity and mystery about consciousness and engages the senses. Organizations can be conscious about change and development, unconscious, or be too wrapped up in the self, precluding consciousness. Gestalt recognizes consciousness in dreams and imagination as sources for creativity and innovation. There are states of consciousness being studied and researched across many disciplines of medicine, sciences, the social sciences, religion and spirituality. Consciousness can exist when an individual's subjective experience of the world results from brain activity. With each experience being different for each organization, two experiences can never be exactly the same.

It answers the questions, "What is happening in the inner and outer world of the system?" and "What is important to understand and pay attention to be successful in the organization's transformation process?" Consciousness requires us to be open-minded to what is and what is not. It is the knowing and not knowing and the knowing unknowing that informs reality in the individual and organization. Consciousness occurs before awareness.

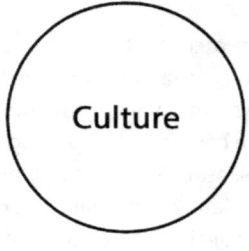

Culture is growing in its importance in the health, well-being, effectiveness, productivity and w/holism of systems. Culture continues to have multiple definitions about "what it is" and "how it is valued". It is fundamental in that it embodies the space for expanding and constricting the success and permeability of boundaries. Culture is often unspoken and unconscious and, at the same time, requires intention and attention in dialogue to surface, thereby bringing clarity to the system. It answers the questions, "What defines, builds and sustains the existence and success of the system (individual, group or organization)"? and "What really matters most to fully commit to as a part of the system"?

Edgar Schein (1997) provides a comprehensive model on organizational culture.

Beyond its schematic clarity, he creates an extended perspective of cultural layers with Artifacts, Espoused Values and Basic Underlining Assumptions. Gestalt helps the practitioner and the client to have clear boundaries and be grounded in the "real self". The answers support the "doing self" and the risk it takes to grow and change. The invisible becomes visible and new behaviors and actions are possible.

A Framework for OD and Change: Three C's

Figure 1. Expanding the C's for Change: Capacity, Capability and Competency

The second set of C's represent the process of development and include capacity, competency and capability. The Heifetz (2003) metaphor would recognize these figures as "being on the dance floor" although they occasionally move to the balcony. These C's are technical challenges and signify levels of expertise, challenges that are significant in their value for achieving performance and organizational results. These words are often seen with an adjective to describe them, such as building capacity, developing competence and creating capability. Frequently, these three C's are used interchangeably with shared and overlapping meanings assigned to them. In many situations, one of the three words is actually used to define one of the other two. It confuses the meaning making and affects the outcome and results. Holding separate and distinct meanings for each C concept increases its individual strength and its contribution to the whole.

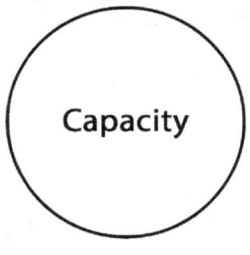

Capacity can be described as a boundary or a container that defines the organization as an entity and holds the organization's current and future potential. It answers the questions, "Who are I /we today?" and "Who do I/we want to be in the future?" Capacity offers the broadest view of what is possible and defines what the organization can live up to in terms of its fit with its stated purpose and its ability to have an impact in the world. Whether an organization focuses globally and/or locally, capacity determines its reach and operational boundaries, the scope of its current work and actions, and the strategic possibilities that could become the shape of its future.

At the core of capacity are the organization's mission, vision and values – what the organization is in business to do, and what drives and guides how it goes about doing it. Capacity has to do with what Collins and Porras (2002) refer to as "clock building" (i.e., building a great organization that will thrive and prosper over time around a "core value system" and ideology) rather than "time telling" (e.g., relying on one great product idea or a charismatic leader as wholly responsible for the organization's success over time, or paying too much attention to profit to the exclusion of everything else).

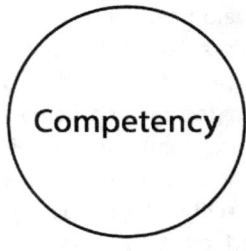

Competency is a critical aspect of an organization's business strategy and a major contributing factor to its success. The components of organizational competency emphasized in this model include the knowledge, skills, attributes, mindsets, and behaviors of the organization's human resources, all of which are required to accomplish its mission, develop strategies to maintain and improve its competitive position, and ensure its long-term sustainability. Competency answers the questions, "What do we know?" and "What can we do?"

Each individual, group, and the organization itself has a core set of competencies that are significant assets in helping the organization leverage the strengths of its workforce and outperform its competitors. Competencies can be – and frequently are -- major differentiators for both individuals and organizations when it comes to comparisons and competition in the marketplace.

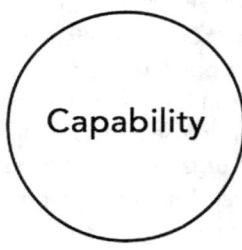

Capability answers the questions, "How are we performing?" and "What are we known for when we are at our best?" Capability helps define what is unique about the organization as it leverages its resources through the work of individuals, teams and groups working across boundaries and in partnership with each other to produce outcomes that add value and achieve the organization's strategic goals. Capability is the result of making clear choices to get the most out of the organization's core sets of competencies as these are applied to the organization's capacity.

Capability capitalizes on asking and answering the right questions to achieve concentrated and motivated results that exceed expectations, strengthen relationships and commitments with customers and employees, and build the organization's reputation for innovative ideas, products and services.

The measurement of capability equates to new learning in vertical development beyond continuous improvement of skills. Improving capability can be directly related to the actual performance of the individual as it relates to the performance of the organization. The capability needs must have clear intentions and focused attentions to competency moving from the expert and achiever development level to be a catalyst for change. Linking the individual's learning to the organization's performance are essential aspects of the growth and future of the organization. For transformational change, capability requires a higher level of awareness. It means challenging basic assumptions, the culture, mindsets and behaviors and creating scalable opportunities for of the organization. It represents to what extent contact is being made in the individual and the system about "what is."

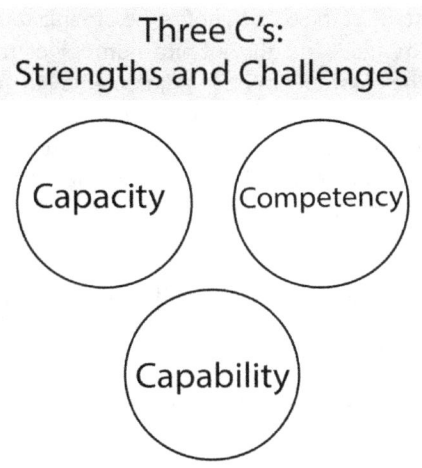

Figure 2. Three C's Strengths and Challenges

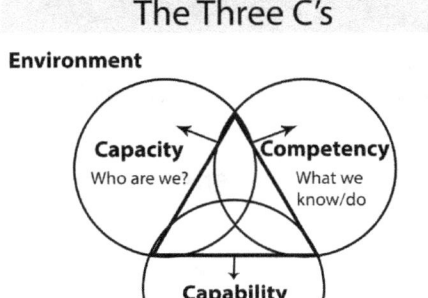

Figure 3. The Second Set of C's Framework with Overlapping Triangle

Making Meaning Leads to New Systemic Patterns

Gestalt practice and System thinking provide organizing principles for working at the organization level of system. Understanding the largest level of system in and of itself is very complex and the development of the system takes an enormous amount of inner and outer collective wisdom and "gutsy will". Gestalt refers to a configuration of patterns and the 6 C's are a set of critical elements in the pattern of a system. Holding the "Gestalt" of the 6 C's benefits the organization as it becomes more aware of its field and the infinite number of realities. Growth occurs when the system makes adjustments in relation to its environment with new ways of being and doing. It must pay attention to its practices such as strategy, execution, structure and innovation. The C's create a framework that helps the organization shift its ground, build common ground and shared figures.

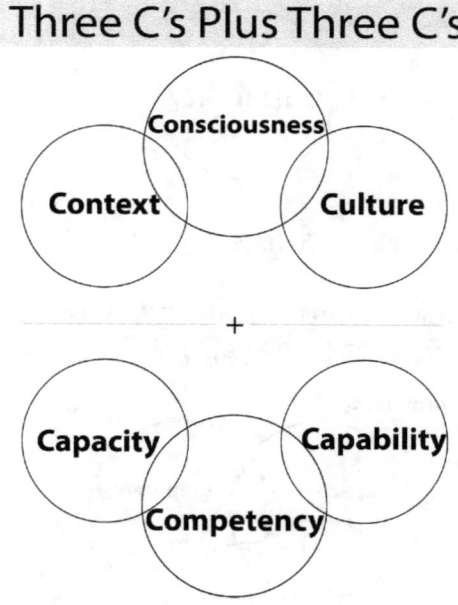

Figure 4. A Gestalt of the 6 C's

The Process of Change and Transformation

Organizations cannot avoid the need for change, and transformation requires deep change. The Gestalt practitioner's work becomes a catalyst for change and transformation and supports the appropriate level of work in organizations, facilitating the organization as a whole to discover the needs and challenges that most excite and motivate. In the meaning making and the differences a Gestalt practitioner can lead organizations through an extensive review of previously unexamined areas to develop new insights about the organization's potential. The engagement can range from engaging with the current reality to understanding the organization's human capital to meeting the challenges the organization is facing. The complexities of this process occur within an ever-changing organizational environment. From new perspectives, actions emerge that result in organizational changes that produce a competitive advantage.

Paradoxes and Change

Paradox 1: *Organizations don't change unless they have to change.*

> As the rate of change increases the organization must have a readiness to respond quickly with new and creative ideas. Organizations do not change easily in a global environment and often the need for changes is not seen, or is missed or ignored. In many situations, forces in the external environment drive the organization's need for change without giving organizations a choice. There is typically a cumulative impact from old ways of thinking, entrenched and outdated behaviors and not having a sense of urgency to face these challenges. Organizations learn that change requires good data, new organizational designs, becoming customer centric and a systems view about a long-term transformation to move towards its new state.

Paradox 2: *Organizations find it increasingly difficult even when they want to make changes to adjust to trends, develop talent and meet growth targets.*

> Organizations are more profit driven and less relational, which means the focus is on talent rather than people and the value shifts from contact to detachment. The culture and internal environment for change is not measured well

and does not carry the worth in the same way as targets and profits. The bottom line becomes the primary focus with short-term goals and objectives. Many organizations want to ignore or work to control internal forces for change and often label them as forces against the change. There is little tolerance for the lengthy process for change and transformation and insufficient buy-in to build passion and momentum.

Paradox 3: *Organizations may be willing to take risks needed for change and still resist accepting the discomfort and pain experienced while moving into the unknown.*

Current studies and observations of organizations find them with a transactional orientation experiencing increasing pressure on traditional business models, major technology shifts, dynamics of internal relationships and the development of their talent. The new world order for organizations requires transformational changes, which activate deep emotions in the organization and anxiety over losing traditional ways of doing business that no longer serve organizational goals. Transformations require deep systemic change that goes beyond algorithms to dialogue and understanding about the emotional impact of change. Within this context, organizations question if this investment will prepare them for the long term.

In the process of excavating deeper purpose and greater understanding, experiencing the intensity of having world-views clash and diving into the discomfort of the unknown, the organization seeks short-term answers and immediate fulfillment. This understanding will require an organization to zoom in and zoom out in the field to constantly adjust perspectives. The two sets of C's help to generate and measure the extent that the change and transformation is occurring while simultaneously being able to integrate with future trends, radical thinking, and strategies. This richness is built in a "deep dive" using the 6 C's framework.

Traditionally many interactions and, therefore, experiences of change, are transactional and incremental in nature. When the need is for transformational change, however, the scope and level of effort involved is far greater. Transformation is more than simply adding information or resources into the container that already exists, as is the case with incremental change. Transformation is about changing the actual form of the container—making it larger, more complex, and more able to deal with multiple demands and uncertainties. This requires the highest level of attention to, and integration of, all of the C's in order to bring about the emergence of a new state of being through a complete shift, or even the death of, the old state of being. It is the process of creating a new configuration of patterns, in other words, a new Gestalt.

Conclusion

Gestalt practice and Systems perspectives help make visible the dynamism of change. They are theories and practices that are descriptive rather prescriptive approaches to addressing transformation initiatives. The 2 sets of C's are not fixed Gestalts, functioning in linear and cyclical configurations. Each set of C's can be the figure at one point and ground at another point in time. The process of formation happens with good awareness, and with contact and integration with the environment. The C's fit Heifetz's metaphor of being on the balcony and the dance floor. In a time of exponential change, the need is to go back and forth between the two to identify new figures.

This chapter poses some useful questions, encourages new thinking about theory, and expands the possible dimensions of change. It is part of a new dialogue, a journeying together in an "archeological dig" of sorts, into a framework that offers possibilities for discovery in exploring both the phenomena and concepts. These concepts emerge from experiences in organizations and in life, and seek to bring further clarity and motivation to the work. It is in the process of deeper exploration with curiosity and in being open to new possibilities that change and transformation can occur.

Successful organizations continuously monitor their internal and external environments, link strategic and operational change efforts, and manage their human capital resources in rapidly changing environments. New discoveries, new inventions, new technologies, new markets, new products, demographic changes in customer and client groups, new regulations, new mores – all of the changes and complexities involved in today's business environment require new ways of thinking and new or better developed competencies in order to be successful at the organizational, group and individual levels.

References

Beisser, A. (1970). *The Paradoxical Theory of Change* in Fagan, J. and Shepherd, I. (eds.) *Gestalt Therapy Now*. New York: Harper.

Brown, T. (2009). *Change by Design: How Design Thinking Transforms Organizations and Inspires Innovation*. New York: HarperCollins

Church, A. and Burke, W. (2018). 'Four Trends Shaping the Future of Organizations and Organization Development.' *OD Practitioner*, (50)4.

Heifetz R. and Laurie D. (2001). 'The Work of Leadership', *Harvard Business Review*. December 2001.

Collins, J. & Porras, J. (2002). *Built to last: Successful habits of visionary company*. New York: HarperCollins.

Ghitulesco, B. (2013). Making change happen: The impact of work context on adaptive and practice behaviors. *Journal of Applied Behavioral Sciences*, 49(2), pp. 206–245.

Heifetz, R. and Lindsky, M. (2002). *Leadership on the Line: Staying Alive Through the Dangers of Leading*. Boston: Harvard Business School Press.

Jones, B. B. (2014). 'A Framework for Change: Capacity, Capability and Competency', in Jones, B. B. and Brazzel, M. (eds.) *The NTL Handbook for Organization Development and Change*, 2nd ed. New York: John Wiley.

Quinn, R. (1996). *Deep change: Discovering the leader within*. San Francisco, CA: Jossey-Bass.

Ramo, J.C. (2010). *The Age of the Unthinkable: Why the New World Disorder Constantly Surprises Us and What We Can Do About It*. Boston: Little, Brown & Company.

McAfee, A. (2013). *Digital Information; We Haven't Seen Anything Yet*. [Online] Available at: https://www.youtube.com/watch?v=az5epl36bbu

Lewin, K. (1936). *Principles of topological psychology*. New York: McGraw-Hill.

Lewin, K., and Cartwright, D. (ed.) (1951). *Field theory in social science*. New York: Harper.

Nevis, E. (1987). *Organizational Consulting: A Gestalt Approach*. New York: Gardner Press.

Perls, F. (1969). *Ego, Hunger and Aggression*. New York: Random House

Petrie N. (2014). Vertical Leadership-Part 1. White Paper. Center for Creative Leadership. Greensboro, North Carolina.

Schein, E. H. (1993). 'On dialogue, culture and organizational learning', *Organizational Dynamics*, 22(2), pp. 40–51.

Ulrich, D., & Smallwood, N. (2004). 'Capitalizing on Capabilities.' *Harvard Business Review*, von Bertalanffy, L. (1988). *General System Theory: Foundations, Development, and Applications, Revised Edition*. New York: Braziller.

Wheeler, G. (1988). *Gestalt Reconsidered: A New Approach to Contact and Resistance*. Cleveland: Gestalt Institute of Cleveland Press.

Yontef G. M. (1993). *Awareness, Dialogue & Process: Essays on Gestalt Theory*. New York: The Gestalt Journal Press, Inc.

Chapter 17: Gestalt in Organizations: Experiences from Practice in West Africa Cultural Underpinnings of Resistances in Organisational Change: Lessons from Gestalt OD Practice in West Africa

John Nkum and Daniel K. B. Inkoom

Overview

The application of Gestalt in organizations is relatively unknown in many of the countries and large public sector organizations in West Africa. In the past decade, however, there has been a steady growth in the number of organisation development practitioners (estimated to be around 150-200[*]) who use the Gestalt body of knowledge in their practice. Many of these practitioners are products of three programs that have trained West Africans in the past 15-18 years. These are the International Organisation and Systems Development Program (IOSD) that was organized from Cleveland, Ohio, and conducted internationally from 1992 till 2012; the Organisation and Systems Development Practitioner Formation Program (OSDPFP) that was offered in Ghana from 2006 to 2013; and the International Gestalt Organisation and Leadership Development (iGOLD) program, offered by GestaltOD partners, an international faculty of Gestalt practitioners from 2012 to date. There is anecdotal evidence that these few GestaltOD practitioners in West Africa are steadily influencing leadership behavior and perceptions in the organizations with which they work by introducing some key principles

---

[*] There is no database of GestaltOD practitioners in West Africa. The estimate comes from the list of participants in the three main programs that have been training West Africans in the application of Gestalt in organizations since 1992.

of Gestalt, such as holism, interconnectedness, use of self and presence, relationship mastery and systems thinking. This trend is likely to grow.

In this chapter, the authors share their practice of GestaltOD in West Africa, drawing attention to how some cultural worldviews and systemic mental constructs that are prevalent in the region enhance or slow down the application of Gestalt in organisational change processes. Using cases from their many years of consulting practice in Ghana, Nigeria, Liberia, and Sierra Leone, the authors seek to map the varied manifestations of resistances in organizations they have supported to go through change and how application of the Gestalt body of knowledge supported the management of those resistances

The authors use the cycle of experience* at the individual and organisational levels as a frame to map their practice in organizations, identifying the emergence of various forms of culturally informed resistances, and the application of Gestalt principles and concepts in the management of these resistances along the cycle. The purpose is to enhance awareness among GestaltOD practitioners in Africa, and share experiences from practice in how to embrace and manage resistances through the application of GestaltOD principles, concepts and models in organizational consulting.

The authors take cases from organizational capacity development and change management programs, individual and team coaching practice, teambuilding and culture change experiences in the public, private and the non-profit sectors. They identify patterns of culturally informed resistances across levels of system, indicating the contexts that inform the resistances, and how the application of GestaltOD enables the management of these resistances to support movement towards the change objectives.

This paper provides snippets and insights from field practice, seeking to broaden the repertoire of responses practitioners in West Africa might deploy in managing resistances in organizational change processes that are steeped in cultural beliefs and perceptions. The mapping of underlying cultural factors to resistances provides awareness to both the GestaltOD consultant and the client system, supporting them to mobilize the appropriate energy towards action and contact. This calls for a good understanding of the cultural context that enables the

---

* As originally presented by John Carter (2008) in Gestalt organisation and systems development and OD; past, present and future perspectives. *OD Practitioner. 40 (4), 49-51*

Gestalt OD practitioner to support emergence in systems and to work in ways that enhance awareness and support change. It also provides perspectives on ways of being and how to energize systems to do effective work at different levels of system. This is significant in a high-power distance, hierarchical and patriarchal cultural context where leadership is perceived as strength and power rather than a results-based and collaborative effort. It is also significant because of the predominant perception and culture of followers in West Africa that they are victims of change, and/or are entitled to good life and services that their leaders must provide. The organizational culture in West Africa presents tensions that may be evident as polarities of: hierarch and victim; agency and entitlement; honor and shame; loyalty and "truth-speaking" to power; wisdom and youthfulness; modernism and cultural traditions; drive and fatalism. These polarities and underlying cultural dynamics underpin various resistances to change in organizations in ways that are not obvious to the uninformed GestaltOD practitioner in West Africa. This paper speaks to these dynamics and how to navigate change in these complex contexts.

The paper also postulates that given the ongoing trends in global development contexts and needs, it is likely that the practice of GestaltOD will become even more popular in West Africa. This calls for a strategic approach that would continuously expose many more professionals to this body of knowledge in ways that support systems to be more effective.

Organisational Change Practices, and Evidence of Resistances

The reflections in this paper are derived from periods of consulting at different levels of system and in different institutions across several countries in West Africa, including Ghana, Liberia, Nigeria and Sierra Leone. In Ghana, the focus was on consulting institutions and individuals in both the public and private space, as well as the not-for profit sector, as well as capacity development in organization development consultancy for second year MBA students of the Business School of the Kwame Nkrumah University of Science and Technology, Kumasi. The interventions in Ghana also included providing short-to medium term organization development support to a wide range of institutions including international and national non-governmental organizations.

In Liberia, the context was to help the country to emerge after the civil war that devastated the country in the 1990s. Organization development support was provided as a capacity development package to assist partners of an International organization as part of the Civil Society and Media Leadership (CSML) Programme. The objective was to provide skills, knowledge and tools to individuals working in the partner organizations in order to support these local organizations to be effective, efficient and healthy. The training programme sought to enhance the ability of participants to influence self, individuals, organizations and large systems by increasing their competence in understanding and working with multiple levels of system; improving skills in recognizing and working with multiple realities; managing resistance to change; using diversity as a resource intervening effectively and conflict transformation. By this training, it was hoped that participants would be able to bring about change in organizations; enlarge their appreciation of organizational culture and differences and enhance competence in influencing organizational systems in a multicultural context. It was hoped that after this training, there would be a community of practitioners who work to empower organizations to contribute to sustenance of peace in Liberia. The period of training spanned from August 2013 to June 2014 and involved six one-week teaching sessions in two cities in Liberia.

In Sierra Leone, the interventions were designed for staff of a development cooperation project on decentralization and it involved two sessions of organization development training in the capital Freetown. The focus was to empower the participants with e skills that will allow them to be change agents in partner institutions and to support the decentralization policy that sought to bring power closer to the grassroots. In all these training programmes. In all these interventions, the cultural context of organisations and the country was a central figure in the training. The training was considered to be highly successful, given the feedback received form the institutions and individuals, reflected in further work that we had to do as consultant OD practitioners. In Liberia for example, further assignments including evaluations of individual programmes were foreseen, but were curtailed due to the outbreak of Ebola. A participant from Liberia had this to say in 2018:

> *"I must admit that much of the knowledge and skills acquired in the organization development training you conducted with the RSC team are being applied in my work here at EDC. For example, I always arrange my tasks into 'smaller units of work'. This has helped me to complete my work in a timely manner,*

thereby meeting needed results and desired performance benchmarks"

In Liberia, the Gestalt Key concept of awareness was also a main theme for the training. It was important, for example, to build into the training, an awareness of how culture can serve as a tool to enable people to become agents of change. Awareness is essentially our experience of our own senses and our bodies in relation to the environment we find ourselves at a particular moment of time. In the Gestalt frame, it can be said to be our own experience in the "Here and now". Dealing with participants from Civil Society Organizations and community radio stations, this theme was used to help participants understand how they could be agents of change in rebuilding the country after the civil war, given the predominant spaces they occupied in society. It was for example important to let participants experience how on the Cycle of Experience, one moves from Sensation to Figure-with-Awareness, which is unfocused, sensory awareness to awareness of the emerging figure. Coming out of war, it was important to help participants notice how we can become aware of "habitual figures" or the tendency towards "fast figures" especially as the country struggled through the process of reconciliation and nation building after the war. The issue of power was also explored in terms of who had the power to effect change after war. It was particularly important to note how the media was used as an agent of change in the post-war period.

"We can be more powerful than the soldiers in bringing about change" was an apt comment by one of the participants from the community radio stations during one of the training sessions. The realization that the airwaves, just as they could be used to propagate war (as in the Rwandan genocide for example) could also be strong agents of change was emphasized, as well as the individual/collective roles in bringing about change. In Liberia at the time of the training, there was the urgent need for the organizations who participated in the training to help foster planned development and change in social systems. This meant that OD fitted into the body of knowledge that could help explain how individuals, groups, organizations, communities, and even societies change and how each of these levels of system are pertinent to the change management process. The OD value of human dignity, respect for the other irrespective of gender, ethnicity and affiliation became prominent in the training development theme.

In Ghana, work at the Business School focused on, among others, the extent of culture as a determinant in the nature and scope of work in institutions and by implication the orientation needed for organization development consulting. As early OD practice focused on "what do I need to learn" as practitioners explored systems to understand and provide support to what was missing in organizations, there was a conscious effort to put emphasis on how educational institutions could become the places where knowledge generation could support OD practice. The opportunity to teach a course in "organization development consulting" was therefore a good opportunity to explore ways of integrating academic knowledge with industrial practice. This frame was deemed important as being a prerequisite for successful OD practice. The work at the University also presented opportunities to shape what forms OD practice could mean, and the scope of OD practice after school, especially in the Ghanaian and West African context where formal organisation development practice is at its formative stages. In spite of the organizational culture of teaching across disciplines, there were overt and covert resistances in having an external resource persons from outside the Business School to facilitate this capacity development. However, these resistances depended on the posture of persons required to take the decisions on who is invited to teach. Where these persons had knowledge of the role of OD consulting or had gone through a period of training themselves, it was much training was easily facilitated. The opposite was also true. In many instances, the Business School was flexible enough to allow the introduction of field experiences from practicing OD professionals, and this greatly enhanced teaching and learning. It was insightful to learn from the evaluation done at the end of these periods of engagement. Much as many students were not sure how avenues would open to them after their course in the field of organisation development consulting, there were a number of cases where classmates teamed up to start consulting on their own, benefitting for the class experiences and coaching which the authors continue to provide, as a process of integrating recent graduates to industry. Above all, students became more aware of the need to pay particular attention to context, because the generally "western orientation" of the educational system in Ghana.

Insights and the Way Forward for OD Practice in West Africa

Hofstede's theory of cultural dimensions exposes the impact of a society's culture on the values, norms and behaviours of its members and the theory has been extensively used in many fields as a model for research particularly in the fields of cross-cultural psychology, international management, and cross-cultural business communication (www.geerthofstede.nl). In the context of West Africa, this theory appears to be of relevance for work in organisations at all level of system. Given the colonial history of many of the countries in West Africa, it is important to reflect on how culture has been embedded in the work place environment and what that means for organisation development and change management. The impact of other cultures as a result of colonization also

Hofstede (2003) argues that if not properly understood, culture is more often a source of conflict than synergy and cultural differences are a nuisance and often a disaster (www.geert-hofstede.com). Hofstede further asserts that despite evidence that people from different cultural backgrounds behave differently, there is the tendency to assume cultural monotony, leading to the minimization of cultural differences and peculiarities. This stance can in turn brew new conflict and entrench existing ones. The Gestalt concept of awareness of these differences was therefore important in order to facilitate development within societies and organisations in the West African context.

The key observation is that as a growing field, the practice of organisation development in West Africa should take into consideration the cultural context within the individual countries and organizations as a prerequisite for effective organisational work and change management. Experiences from the field also indicates the need to continue to build the capacity of professionals in the field of organisation development so as to provide the expertise for the need of industry in the near future. Furthermore. The need to embrace the environment within which cultural practices are influenced by "outside forces" is key for OD practice to evolve fully in West Africa.

Conclusions

"Context is everything" appears to sum up the experiences in West Africa. The particular cultural practices in the case countries calls for a clear understanding from the Gestalt OD intervener to employ approaches that allow the bringing on board and integration of cultural imperatives in OD practice in West Africa. The OD practitioner also has to stay in awareness of the global environment and how cultural practices respond in the face of global influences. It is this stance that will allow OD practice in West Africa to assure its relevance and ability to respond effectively to cultural context of developments now and in the future.

From indications in different levels of system, the OD practitioner has to prepare for the "explosion" of OD practice in West Africa, but must do so with awareness of the cultural context that defines who we are and ways we act. This has to be done conscious of "organism/environment" interactions and how we are changed at the contact boundary with the local and global environment. The OD practice that will be a means to transform society in developmental ways in our context will be one that integrates actors in all levels of system and staying close to the "here and now" to understand what societies and institutions require for the transformation process.

References:

Carter, J. (2008). Gestalt organisation and systems development and OD: past, present and future perspectives. *OD Practitioner. 40(4)*, pp. 49-51.

Hofstede, G. (2003). *Culture's consequences: Comparing values, behaviours, institutions, and organisations across nations*. Thousand Oaks, CA: SAGE Publications.

Hofstede, G. and Minkov, M. (2010). *Cultures of the organisation: Software of the mind*. New York: McGraw-Hill.

Inkoom, D.K.B. (2014). *Training Report in Organisation Development*. Monrovia, Liberia: IREX.

Kwesi, A. S. (2014). *Cultural Diversity and Multiculturallism in Ghanaian Companies* [Online]. Available at: https://www.ghanaweb.com/GhanaHomePage/features/Cultural-Diversity-and-Multiculturalism-in-Ghanaian-Companies-339562 (Accessed: 12 December 2018).

Afterword

Robert J. Marshak

I found the emphasis in this book on wHolism important and it stimulated in me several reflections about the field of organizational change, especially Organization Development (OD), which I wish to share here. Let me first set the context for my comments. I do not consider myself a Gestaltist. I am, of course familiar with Gestalt theory and practice in general, but have not studied it like many of my colleagues who have contributed to this book. Instead I suppose I am a long time practitioner, theorist, educator, and commentator about OD consulting and change. My comments are offered from that context.

For the past decade or so I, like many others, have noticed and commented on the increasing divisions within the fields associated with organizational change, again with particular attention to OD. It seems as if each decade since the 1950s has added a new set of theories and/or methods to what is considered OD. This, in itself, is a sign of a vibrant and growing field. At the same time many of the advocates of the newer approaches touted them as being superior to long established (read outdated) theories and practices. This positioned the various ideas and practices, both new and more established, as competitors more so than allies. Concurrently, those practicing OD moved from the founding generation(s) where addressing social and organizational change was an avocation of scholar-practitioners to later generations where practicing OD had become a vocation in a world where consulting to organizational change was a multi-billion dollar industry. This, combined with the presumed increased competence and attractiveness to potential clients of being a specialist, along with many other factors, has led us to what some call the present state of fragmentation in OD and related change fields. Personally, I have chosen to call it increased differentiation without much integration. The result has been increasingly specialized theories and practices focused on separate domains of organizational or societal change issues, with practitioners joining separate affinity networks and conferences and losing touch and interest with their colleagues in other siloes.

This brings me back to the theme of holism. It strikes me that recent history has promoted addressing specialized aspects of change or change issues rather than working from more holistic perspectives. Might, therefore, "holism," the consideration of the dynamics and interdependencies of the total situation, become one possible integrating theme? Including holism as an essential core to the practice of organizational change would be a call to insist that practitioners be adept at being able to help clients deal with issues and opportunities from a total systems perspective. This in turn would ask practitioners to broaden their range of theories and practices while also learning what the "holism perspective in organizational change" means and what ways of thinking and doing are associated with it. Now, I imagine, my Gestalt readers at this point are thinking, "That's what Gestalt is and that's what we do!" Before I comment on that directly let me raise a few considerations.

First, let's go back to Kurt Lewin, a Berlin School trained Gestaltist, who also is widely considered to be the source of virtually all the seminal ideas in social change and what later became known as the field of OD. His iconic three stage model of change (*unfreeze-movement- freeze*), action research, democratic principles, and the like, helped launch a process-oriented, humanistic approach to social and organizational change that still resonates for most OD and other change practitioners. To my way of thinking, however, in today's increasingly specialized and differentiated world of change theory and practice another core aspect of his contributions has been diminished over time. That aspect is his Field Theory and specifically that behavior results from the dynamics of the total field of experience. For Lewin this foregrounded holism in change theory and practice: interdependencies, relationships, and the consideration of the total context of internal and external factors and forces. How ironic that a legacy that began with holism as a central concept is now dealing with fragmentation and concerns about a lack of integration within an increasingly differentiated field of theories and practices.

Next, let me comment briefly on Gestalt psychology and organizational change. Gestalt psychology predates OD and both have developed in parallel over the past 60 years or so. Within that time period significant institutes, programs, writings, theories and practices that specifically apply Gestalt thinking to organizational and social change have emerged. Some would call those applications "Gestalt OD" and, like the chapters in this book, they advocate holistic approaches to consulting and change. In that regard Gestalt OD may well represent a truer version of Lewin's original total system core principle than many contemporary OD practices. Here, then, is an integrating theme that I believe is needed across the many approaches to OD and social change and it already exists in theory as well as practice. All that is well and good from my point of view.

There is, however, another difficulty to contend with. That difficulty is twofold. The first part is the degree to which Gestalt approaches to consulting and change incorporate disciplines and thinking beyond psychology. And, for that matter whether or not practitioners and potential clients associate such approaches with something more than just psychology and "people-related" issues. Gestalt, of course means holism, but is widely known as a school of psychology to most everyday people (if known at all). As a result, Gestalt OD for many means a type of "psychological OD" that presumably is especially helpful when dealing with a certain range of issues, but not others. This contributes to the second part of the difficulty. That is that "Gestalt OD", at least in my experience, is viewed by many involved in change consulting to be still another separate specialization. Once again, how ironic that an approach to consulting and change centrally based on holism is considered by many to be a separate (and competing) specialization.

All these reflections about the current state of organizational change approaches, especially OD, triggered by the title and writings in this book, lead me to several afterword thoughts:

1. Holistic thinking and acting in OD and other change approaches need to be more centrally positioned and elaborated than is the current case.
2. Holism as an acknowledged central aspect of all OD approaches would also provide at least one integrating mechanism for a presently highly differentiated field.
3. Current Gestalt-oriented theorists and practitioners may need to incorporate a broader range of disciplines and change issues to move beyond being considered a type of psychological specialist.
4. More foregrounding of holism and what it means would be helpful to practitioners and clients alike.

The ideas and insights provided by the authors of the chapters in this book suggest that at least among them these ideas are already being modeled and put into practice. In that regard I hope this book will stimulate in its readers new ways of thinking about organizational consulting and change that perhaps go beyond their current ideas and practices. And, finally I hope my invitation to further advance holism as a central concept for everyone involved in organizational change is accepted by all of the book's readers, authors and editors.

Gestalt Glossary of Theory, Principles, Models and Terms

Action. Phase of the Cycle of Experience where energy is mobilized and there is movement toward fulfilling a need, desire, or goal. The client has a level of excitement and willingness to relax boundaries and borders in order to engage with self, with other or with the broader environment.

Awareness. Phase in the Cycle of Experience where Gestalts and figures form after sensing, scanning and data collection. Because awareness is a natural part of human experience, one can be both consciously and unconsciously aware. The Gestalt practitioner works to be more consciously aware and to heighten the awareness of the client. Thus, awareness is consciously knowing in the moment, mindfulness, and cognizance. Awareness is the centerpiece of Gestalt practice and places emphasis on the "here and now."

Bracketing. The practitioner's intentional focus on avoiding the imposition of personal values, attitudes, beliefs and behaviors in order to provide professional and ethical support to clients.

Boundary (Border). Visible and invisible line of demarcation and separation that establishes limits of interaction among subparts of a social system or between a system and its environment. Boundaries provide definition and identity and can be open or closed; thick or thin; narrow or wide; deep or shallow; near or far. The boundary between self and environment must be sufficiently permeable to allow for exchanges, yet firm enough to enable autonomous thinking and action. Dysfunctional disturbance occurs when the boundary is impermeable, unclear, or lost. Boundaries both limit and liberate.

Closure. Phase of the Cycle of Experience that supports the natural tendency for experiences to finish and be complete. May include actually finishing or completing, and when not possible, acknowledging what remains unfinished or incomplete. The process of closure involves (1) review of goals achieved, (2) assimilation of learning, and (3) identification of next steps. A role of the Gestalt intervener is to facilitate good closure.

Contact. Phase of the Cycle of Experience that is the place of change, transformation, shift, and new learning. It is characterized by mutual exchange of energy across a boundary/border between parts of the organism, an organism and a different organism, or the organism and its environment. The organism is different after genuine (versus pseudo) contact. Contact is a crucial step toward transformation.

Creative Indifference or Void or Point of Balance. Concept developed by expressionist philosopher Salomon Friedlander describing the place from which the differentiation into opposites takes place. He explained that since all existing things are determined by polarities, the zero point (place of suspended judgment) holds the greatest hope for how the world deals with difference. The basic assumption is that the split that man creates in the world through his consciousness, you/me, up/down, black/white, poor/rich, east/west is merely an illusion and can only be eliminate by understanding the world from a zero or neutral position – the no-thing point, the absolute, the origin.

Cycle of Experience. The Gestalt descriptive model, the Cycle of Experience is a blueprint for tracking need satisfaction through the stages of sensation, awareness, energy, action, contact, closure, and withdrawal. Early conceptual perspective came from Kurt Lewin in his field theory on the relationship between a person in the "field," later depicted as a process by Fritz Perls, and refined as a visual model at the Gestalt Institute of Cleveland. The Cycle of Experience is primarily used to track follow naturally occurring, here and now phenomena.

Dream Work. The client is asked to write down their dream with full details, enlisting every person in the dream – the event, weather, mood, every possible detail. Each detail is assumed to be the client's projection of self. The client is asked to prepare a script of conversations between different characters in his dream.

Empty Chair (Experiment in Gestalt practice). A role-play where the client engages in a conversation to understand different aspects of a conflict, experience, issue, or themselves. The practitioner arranges two chairs face to face. The client sits in each chair alternately, expressing only the side of the conflict that is represented by the chair where he is sitting, thereby, creating a verbal dialogue of his feelings. The purpose is to gain insights by bringing to the "here and now" unfished business, an important interaction that is forthcoming or conflict with another individual.

Exaggeration Exercise (Experiment in Gestalt practice). Involves either the practitioner exaggerating the behaviors, gestures or some other traits of the client or the client exaggerating themselves to heighten awareness of their true feelings. During the experiment, the client is asked to repeat or exaggerate a particular behavior, expression, or moment, such as frowning, tapping their foot on the floor, saying repeatedly "I will achieve my goals" to experience the emotion attached to the behavior.

Existentialism. A tradition of philosophical thinking associated mainly with the 19th and 20th century that deals with human existence. Existentialists believe philosophy should begin at the human level – the feeling, behaving, living person – not merely the thinking level. Many existentialists regarded traditional systematic or academic philosophies, both style and content, as too abstract and remote from concrete human experience. Gestalt work is existential in its orientation.

Experiment in Gestalt practice. An experiential learning tool that is distinct in its bias toward action in the moment. The Gestalt practitioner encourages and supports the client to try something new "in the moment" to increase learning and expand options. This is different from an exercise in that an experiment is tailored and designed to the client situation in the here-and-now. Experiments are deemed "safe emergencies" because they attempt to respond to emergent issues that may be experienced as risky under the skilled guidance and support of an intervener. Principles of experiment can be used to design pilot programs as part of planned change initiatives. Examples of experiments in Gestalt therapy are language, dialogue such as Empty Chair, and fantasy.

Fertile Void. A state of being where nothing is standing out or attracting interest, where there is no direction to energy.

Figure/Ground. A type of perceptual grouping which is a vital necessity for recognizing objects through vision. In Gestalt psychology, a "figure" that is foreground is distinguished from the "ground" that is background. The human perceptual tendency is to separate whole figures from their backgrounds based on one or more of a number of possible variables, such as contrast, color, size, etc. A simple composition may have only one figure. In a complex composition, there will be several figures to notice. As we look from one thing to another, they each become figure in turn and we may need to choose an "uppermost figure."

Force Field. In the social sciences, a concept created by Gestalt psychologist Kurt Lewin that provides a framework for looking at the factors (forces) that influence a social situation. Force Field analysis looks at forces that are either driving movement toward a goal (helping forces) or blocking movement toward a goal (hindering forces).

Gestalt [gəˈʃtaːlt] The operational principle of Gestalt psychology which loosely translated means unified whole. Refers to the configuration or pattern of a set of elements. Essence and shape of an entity's complete or whole form that is different and distinct from the sum of its parts.

International Gestalt Organization and Leadership Development (iGOLD). A Gestalt approach to organization, leadership and large social system development and change. The iGOLD perspective is a holistic and integrated stance that addresses and includes a complex mix of social, political, cultural, economic and technological dynamics. The iGOLD perspective is a unique blend of classic OD and change theory, Gestalt theory and Gestalt therapeutic practice, general systems theory, and leadership theory, making it possible to work with individuals, pairs, trios, groups, organizations and larger social systems.

Gestalt Prayer. The 56-word quotation by Fritz Perls that gained attention in popular culture in the 1960s. It describes his thoughts about how life should be lived.

> *I do my thing and you do your thing.*
>
> *I am not in this world to live up to your expectations,*
> *and you are not in this world to live up to mine.*
> *You are you, and I am I,*
> *and if by chance we find each other, it's beautiful.*
> *If not, it can't be helped.*
>
> (Fritz Perls, *Gestalt Therapy Verbatim*, 1969)

The meaning of the Gestalt prayer encourages the individual to live according to their own needs and what feels right instead of looking to outside influences. The statements also emphasize the fact that when individuals are fulfilled, they are better able to help others to do the same, leading to stronger relationships.

Gestalt Psychology or Gestaltism. A theory of mind and brain of the Berlin School that maintains that the brain is holistic, parallel, and analogous with self-organizing tendencies. This Gestalt principle asserts that the human eye sees objects in their entirety before perceiving their individual parts, suggesting the whole is different than the sum of its parts. Secondarily, the whole is anticipated and even sought when the parts are not integrated or complete.

Gestalt Therapy. An existential/experiential form of psychotherapy that focuses on personal responsibility, client experience in the moment, the therapist-client relationship, the broader context of the client's situation, and the client's response to their life's situation. Rather than aiming to move the client to be different, the Gestalt therapist accepts clients as they are and using increased awareness of the here and now to promote health, growth and development. Founded by Fritz Perls, Laura Perls, Isadore From and Paul Goodman in the 1940s. The Perls' had worked with Kurt Goldstein, who applied principles of Gestalt psychology to neurosis. Laura Perls studied with Gestalt psychologists at Berlin University before becoming a psychoanalyst and before working to develop Gestalt therapy. Gestalt therapy is not the same as Gestalt psychology though Gestalt psychology influenced the development of Gestalt therapy.

Holism. A philosophical concept built on the assumption that natural systems (physical, biological, chemical, social, economic, mental, linguistic, etc.) and their properties should be viewed as wholes, not as collections of parts. This often includes the view that systems function as wholes and their functioning cannot be fully understood solely in terms of their component parts. The term *holism* was coined in 1926 by South Africa statesman Jan Smuts. It is derived from Ancient Greek *holos* ὅλος, meaning «all, whole, entire, total." and was coined by.

Homeostasis. The property of a system that regulates its internal environment in an effort to maintain a stable, relatively constant condition.

Intervention. An action intended to influence behavior, emotional state or feelings. In Gestalt practice, an intervention is used to increase the client's self-awareness and foster healthy emotions, attitudes and habits and improve the client's interaction with others and the environment.

Life space. From Kurt Lewin's field theory that states that each person exists in a psychological field or "life space." Lewin theorized that an individual has multiple life spaces. Life space can also be applied to a group or larger system.

Making the Rounds (Experiment in Gestalt Therapy). The client is asked to go to each person in the group and talk to them. Every round has its own theme, for example, self-worth, physical appearance, competence. For example, the client may be given the task to go to each person and say to them "I am competent." It helps when client s talk to others, defend themselves, confront others and disclose themselves.

Multiple realities. All participants in a system hold their individual perceptions and realities by virtue of their different driving needs and experiences. The GOLD perspective considers all perceptions as valid, valuable data, worthy of acknowledgement and use in a consulting or leadership process. Surfacing multiple realities is an integral part of the work of a Gestalt intervener.

Optimism. Gestalt holds to the organismic integrity of the human organism, striving to function optimally in the circumstances in which it finds itself. A philosophical tenet of Gestalt work relates to the drive towards self-actualization of the human organism, an inherently optimistic approach that holds that every person or system is "doing the best they can at any given moment" in the circumstances in which they find themselves.

Organism/Environment (O/E). Each and every living organism has its specific surrounding medium of environment with which it continuously interacts and remains fully adapted. The environment is the sum total of physical and biotic conditions influencing the responses of the organism. The study of the relationship between an organism and its environment is called Ecology.

Kurt Lewin, Gestalt psychologist, believed neither nature (inborn tendencies) nor nurture (how life experience shape individuals) account for human behavior, rather both nature and nurture interact to shape each person. He expressed the relationship between the person and environment in behavioral terms as the formula, $B = f(P, E)$. This is translated as behavior is a function of the person and the environment. Lewin referred to the adjacent space between person and environment as the "boundary zone."

Fritz Perls, co-founder of Gestalt therapy commented, "No individual is self-sufficient; the individual can exist only in an environmental field.

GESTALT GLOSSARY OF THEORY, PRINCIPLES, MODELS AND TERMS

The individual is inevitably, at every moment, a part of some field. His behavior is a function of the total field, which includes both him and his environment."

Organization Development. A collaborative effort between consultant and client for improving the overall effectiveness of an organization using methods of applied behavioral science. OD took shape during the sensitivity and T-group movement that began in the late 1950s.

Paradoxical Theory of Change. Created by Arnold Beisser in 1970, states that change begins not by attending to the future state of "what might be" but by attending to the present state of "what is now." The future can happen when the present is embraced.

Perceived Weirdness Index (PWI). Interveners need to be different enough to model and add value, but not so different as to be repelled by the system.

Perception. The way humans organize and interpret sensations and make sense and meaning of everything in the environment.

Phenomenology. A philosophical perspective that concentrates on the study of consciousness and direct experience. Gestalt places emphasis on immediate experience and raw sensory data in the moment, untainted by meaning, interpretation, or judgment.

Pragnanz. The perceptual process described by Max Wertheimer, Czech psychologist and a founder of Gestalt psychology. Perceiving in simplest forms or wholes, before or in parallel to taking in the individual parts.

Presence. Gestalt practitioners use their presence to support learning and change in others. Presence is defined as the distinctive use of self that is created by the integration of all elements of the practitioner – affection, perception, cognition, behavior – that is interesting enough to the client to achieve and maintain a learning and development partnership. Presence begins with how the practitioner shows up (values, beliefs, dress, points of view, etc.).

With presence, the intervener seeks to provide what is missing in the client system and model what is possible. Presence is intentional, compelling yet non-charismatic.

Resistance. Force that interrupts, challenges, or opposes movement toward a desired goal, whether intentionally or unintentionally executed. Gestalt is recognized for its distinct approach to resistance, seeing it as a healthy manifestation of multiple realities and needs in different directions. Gestalt resistances, also known as contact styles, include projection, retroflection, introjection, deflection, desensitization, confluence and egotism.

Reversal Technique (Experiment in Gestalt Therapy). Involves asking the client to do something they have never done before or do something that is completely out of character.

Self-awareness. The capacity and ability to know and recognize oneself as an individual separate from other individuals and the environment.

Sensation. Phase of the Cycle of Experience that refers to the process of sensing our environment through touch, taste, sight, sound, and smell. This information is sent to the brain in raw form/data where perception comes into play.

Systems Theory. It was under the guidance of biologist Ludwig von Bertalanffy in the 1930s that a "general systems" theory emerged that linked both hard and soft sciences. This theory sought to describe the complexity of nature and the world by using a common set of characteristics and terms. Instead of reducing an entity to the sum of its parts, general systems theory emphasized the relationship among the parts and their connection to the whole and broader environment.

Theme. A distinct, recurring, and unifying quality or idea, providing a single distinct character or subject. Theming is an act of recognizing patterns in experience, then bounding and labeling that experience so that it becomes information. In Gestalt practice, a theme holds polarities; ambivalence; conflicting forces of help and hindering forces, push, pull. The Gestalt practitioner can look for the theme in the polarities or look for the polarity in the theme.

Top Dog/Under Dog (Experiment in Gestalt Therapy). An expression coined by Fritz Perls to describe the way people manipulate and torture themselves to avoid healthy contact with their environment.

The *top dog* describes the part of an individual which makes demands based on the idea that the individual should adhere to certain societal norms and standards. The demands are often characterized by «shoulds» and «oughts." The *underdog* describes the part of an individual that makes excuses explaining why the demands should not be met. It is often the case that these excuses are actually acts of internal sabotage to ensure that the demands are never met.

The therapist guides the client through an exercise where the practitioner is asked to take on both of these roles to help the individual develop a healthier relationship with the environment.

Unit of Work. The Gestalt OD planned change model that is used to organize and design processes of change. A unit of work proceeds in three phases that are aligned with the Cycle of Experience: (1) Beginning (sensation, awareness), (2) Middle (mobilization of energy, action, contact/change) and (3) End (closure, withdrawal). A finished unit of work is a clearly bounded, coherent, and understandable experience, project, event, or initiative.

Withdrawal. Phase of the Cycle of Experience that indicates movement through the Cycle is finished and complete for now or permanently. Energy and interest in the situation begin to recede and moves to the background. Time is allowed for rest and pause. The intervener works with the client to let go and move on to other matters.

Zeigarnik Effect. Named after Lithuanian psychiatrist and Kurt Lewin protégé Bluma Zeigarnik. One famous study conducted by Zeigarnik found that individuals remember for a longer period of time the unfinished parts of a task than they remember the finished parts. Lewin explained that psychological tension or energy is retained in the unfinished situation and causes the task to be remembered. Once finished and resolved, the situation recedes from memory. The findings were pivotal because they confirmed Lewin's theory of psychodynamics and led to his now famous field theory.

Collected Biographies

Paul Barber

Paul has served as professor at the Metanoia Institute, as visiting professor at Middlesex University, and as fellow of the Roffey Park Management Institute. A former practicing psychiatric nurse, he established therapeutic communities and co-created programs in therapeutic community practice. He has trained facilitators and been in private practice as a psychotherapist, group facilitator, organizational consultant, and coach for more than 30 years. He is the author of several books including *Becoming a Practitioner Researcher* and *Facilitating Change in Groups and Teams: A Gestalt Approach to Mindfulness*.

Peter Block

Peter Block (Yale University) is an author and citizen of Cincinnati, Ohio. He is founder of Designed Learning, a training company that offers workshops designed to build the skills outlined in his books. He is author of Flawless Consulting, Stewardship, Community, and others. Peter is part of the Economics of Compassion Initiative of Cincinnati and a member of his local neighborhood council. He serves on the board of LivePerson, a provider of online engagement solutions. His work is in the restoration of the common good and creating a world that reclaims our humanity from the onslaught of modernism.

W. Warner Burke

Warner is the Edward Lee Thorndike Professor of Psychology and Education. He is also Editor of the Journal of Applied Behavioral Science. Professor Burke earned his B.A. from Furman University and his M.A. and PhD from the University of Texas, Austin. Prior to coming to TC in 1979, he served in senior positions at Clark University, the NTL Institute, and as executive director of the OD Network. Professor Burke's consulting experience has been with a variety of organizations in business-industry, education, government, religious, and medical systems. A Diplomate in I/O psychology through the American Board of Professional Psychology, he is also a Fellow of the Academy of Management, the Society of Industrial and Organizational Psychology, and past editor of both Organizational Dynamics and The Academy of Management Executive.

Mee-Yan Cheung-Judge

Mee-Yan (PhD) is a "scholar-educator-practitioner" in the field of OD. She is a senior visiting Fellow of Roffey Park Institute, UK and the Singapore Civil Service College. She started and held the dean role in the NTL ODC programme in Europe for 11 years. She is the author of various OD articles, books and reports. She was the recipient of two Life Time Achievement Awards (ODN, 2013; IODA, 2016) for her outstanding contribution to the field of OD globally. HR Magazine in the UK voted her as the number one top influential thinker in September 2018.

Kate Cowie

Kate (BA, Post-graduate, Bristol Business School) is author of *Finding Merlin: a handbook for the human development journey in our new organisational world* (2012). She is a Member of The NTL Institute for Applied Behavioral Science, and the founding Editor of its practitioner's journal, *Practising Social Change*. She established the European Chapter of the Organization Development Network, and leads the Wicked Company network of social change professionals who are committed to the growth of self and others in organisations. She lives in Aberdeenshire, UK.

Gudrun Frank

Gudrun (PhD) is a mechanical engineer based in Germany and a factory planner who knows her trade from the manufacturing on up and into to the management boardrooms. She is the founder of Exprobico, a certified Member of WEConnect International. Her experiences as an international consultant inspired her to develop an innovative competence check. She teaches as an honorary Professor of HR and Entrepreneurship. She presents herself as a Gestalt practitioner. She is member of various research boards.

Jonno Hanafin

Jonno (MBA) is an internationally recognized Gestalt-based organizational change practitioner with 45 years' experience on six continents. He is a trusted advisor to CEOs and Boards focusing on executive transitions, senior team development and culture change in complex systems. Jonno is a thought leader and keynote speaker who emphasizes individuals, groups and organizations exploiting their awareness to learn from their experience. He has been a leader for 35 years in developing change leaders and consultants utilizing a Gestalt perspective.

Jonno is a co-founder of the International Organization & Systems Development (OSD) Program, the international Gestalt Organization & Leadership Development (iGOLD) Program and the iGOLD Center. .

Walt Hopkins

Walt writes, works with groups, and keeps learning – with a focus on human interaction, influencing, and life designing. Walt joined NTL in 1983. He has two diplomas from the Gestalt Institute of Cleveland – in addition to his B.A., M. Litt., and PhD Over the past fifty years, Walt has worked with thousands of people from more than sixty countries, in organisations ranging from Apple to the European Space Agency to the UN World Food Programme.

Daniel K.B. Inkoom

Dan K. B. Inkoom (Dr.rer.pol) graduated from the International Organisation & Systems Development (IOSD) Program in 2004 and is currently Associate Professor of Planning and OD Practitioner at the Kwame Nkrumah University of Science and Technology in Kumasi, Ghana. External examiner to Universities in Ghana, South Africa, Sweden, Tanzania, and Zimbabwe, Daniel was recently appointed visiting Professor at the University of the Witwatersrand in Johannesburg, South Africa for a term ending in 2021.

Brenda B. Jones

Brenda, (MSc) is an Organizational consultant based in the USA with consulting projects in the Americas, Asia, Africa, Europe and the Middle East. She is President of The Lewin Center, on faculty of the American University Key Executive Leadership Development Program and past president of the NTL Institute and the AU/NTL Masters Program in OD.

Brenda received the OD Network's Lifetime Achievement Award in 2012. She is co-editor of The NTL Handbook for Organization Development and Change (2014, 2nd edition). She can be reached at brendabjones1@verizon.net.

Carolyn J. Lukensmeyer

Carolyn (PhD) is Executive Director Emerita of the National Institute for Civil Discourse, an organization working to reduce political dysfunction and incivility in the United States political system. She aims to restore democracy to the intended vision of the founding fathers. Carolyn previously served as Founder and President of America*Speaks*, an award-winning nonprofit organization that promoted nonpartisan initiatives to engage citizens and leaders. She also served as consultant to the USA White House Chief of Staff and on the National Performance Review. She was Chief of Staff in the Ohio Governor's office, becoming the first woman to serve in this capacity.

Ollie Malone Jr.

Ollie is president and principal consultant of Olive Tree Associates. He has headed training and OD functions within Pennzoil-Quaker State, Sprint, and The Mead Corporation. In addition, he has worked as an external consultant with a number of Fortune 500 companies. His more than 20 years' corporate experience also include key roles in marketing, finance, and operations.

He holds degrees (B.A., M.S., MBA, PhD, and D. Min.) in communication, business, education, organization change and development, and transformational leadership. He also completed multiple programs at the Gestalt Institute of Cleveland.

Based in Plano, TX, he is married to Patricia, the father of Nathan, and grandfather to four granddaughters.

Robert J. Marshak

Robert (PhD) is an award winning author, educator and consultant. He is currently distinguished scholar in residence emeritus at American University and maintains a global consulting practice. Bob is known for his pioneering work on dialogic organization development, covert processes in organizational change, East Asian change philosophy, and the use of metaphors and symbolic meaning in organizational change. A chapter about him and his work is included in *The Palgrave Handbook of Organizational Change Thinkers*.

Joseph Melnick

Joseph (PhD) is a Clinical and Organizational Psychologist. He is co-chair of the Cape Cod Training Program and Board Member of the Gestalt International Study Center. The founding editor of *Gestalt Review*, he has authored more than 100 publications, including *Mending the World: Social Healing Interventions by Gestalt Practitioners Worldwide*, (Melnick, and Nevis, E., Eds., 2012), and *The Evolution of the Cape Cod Model*, (Melnick and Nevis, S., 2018). He trains and teaches worldwide.

Eugenio Moliní

Eugenio is a consultant in systemic transformation and organizational resilience. He specialises in the design, facilitation and management of transformational processes in which success depends on collaboration between parties with different perspectives, professions, cultures and even diverging interests. With offices in Madrid and Stockholm, his global practice has served national, multinational and global companies, and international, multilateral, national and local organizations in Sweden and Spain, Africa and Latin America since 1990.

In addition to his consulting practice, Eugenio launched GAIT – "Guild of Agents for Intentional Transformation," a network of people committed to support each other, with the purpose of increasing the impact of their interventions.

Edwin C. Nevis

Edwin co-founded the Gestalt-oriented organizational consulting and management approach.

Edwin taught many years at Massachusetts Institute of Technology (MIT) and held a PhD in Organizational Psychology. Edwin had more than e 40 years of experience advising countless well-known global companies. He also shaped a large international network of Gestalt practitioners. He co-founded the Gestalt Institute of Cleveland, the Gestalt Organization & Leadership (OSD) Program, the Gestalt International OSD Program, and served as editor of the Gestalt Review.

John Nkum

John Nkum (MSc) has over 30 years international consulting experience in process facilitation, organization and leadership development, and change management processes, including multi-stakeholder dialogue processes and executive coaching for many national and international development agencies and corporate bodies. He is the founder and Executive Director of Nkum Associates, a consulting firm, and the Organization Development Centre-Ghana, a non-profit entity, providing consultancy services and training in Gestalt OD. John is also a founding partner of the iGOLD program.

Mary Ann Rainey

Mary Ann (PhD) is a behavioral scientist, executive coach and consultant with a global client base. Her leadership experience includes corporate

Vice-president and Vice-city Manager. Her work in Gestalt involves international co-chairperson roles and co-founder of the International Gestalt Organization & Leadership Development (iGOLD®) Program. Her teaching includes Adjunct Faculty in the Executive MBA Program at Loyola University Chicago, faculty in the Strategic Agility and Innovation Program sponsored by Yale School of Management and Yale New Haven Hospital, and Dean of the NTL OD Certificate Programme UK. She has numerous publications.

Eva Roettgers

Eva (M.A.Paed) has facilitated change and developmental processes for individuals, teams and organizations for over 30 years. She works internationally with a variety of organizations: profit- and non-profit companies, universities and professional associations and is co-founder of IGOR – Institute of Gestalt Organizational Consulting. In the last two years the main focus of her work has been supporting processes to reduce hierarchical structures and powers and increasing openness and capabilities of individuals and organizations for self-organizing, agile team work.

Dorothy E. Siminovitch

Dorothy (PhD, MCC) is an international leadership, team, and organizational coach, mentor coach, speaker, and author. Dorothy is Director of Training for the Gestalt Coaching Program in Istanbul and Toronto, and co-founder and co-owner of the Gestalt Center for Coaching. Dorothy is the author of *A Gestalt Coaching Primer: The Path Toward Awareness IQ*, and co-author of Awareness 20/20™, a leadership awareness instrument grounded in Dorothy's innovative work on presence and use of self.

Chantelle Wyley

Chantelle (MIS) is a South African with a background in anti-apartheid work, community development and development management. Since taking the International Organization & Systems Development (IOSD) Program (1995-6) she has applied Gestalt theory and practice in contexts of socio-economic change, transformation and democratisation in Africa. Chantelle is a co-founder and on the faculty of the International Gestalt Organization and Leadership Development (iGOLD) Program. She is accredited as a Gestalt Practitioner in Organisations (GPO) by the European Association of Gestalt Therapy (EAGT).

Index

Action 253
Action research 42, 44, 250
Adult learning 227
Agile mindset 81, 85, 90
Ambiguity 47, 79, 109, 113, 117–18, 225
Aristotle 11, 94
Authenticity 29, 32, 43, 45, 52, 111, 113
Awareness 34, 43, 45, 61, 62–3, 84, 94, 109–22 *passim*, 123, 132–6, 153–4, 170, 177, 226, 229–30, 242, 245
    Awareness agents 62
    Awareness Model of Change 214–15
    Bound awareness 62–3

Barber, Paul xviii, 27, 262
Beckhard, Richard 17, 18
Beisser, Arnold 94, 100, 259
Berlin School of Gestalt Psychology 42, 250, 257
Best practice xv, 186, 194, 219
Block, Peter xiv, 262
Boundary (Border) xii, 44, 52, 62–3, 78–81, 119, 170, 176, 180, 211
Bracketing 253
Brain, The 60, 77, 79–80, 95, 99, 127, 148, 174, 229, 257, 260
Brentano, Franz 41–2
Bridges, William 15, 21
British Airways 23–4
Buber, Martin 42, 44, 45, 48
Buechner, Frederick 121
Burke, W. Warner xviii, 11, 20, 24, 262

Capability 232
Capacity 231
Carter, John viii, ix, x, 212, 214, 242
Case Western Reserve University 5, 64
Change 59, 77, 79, 94, 109, 157, 168, 169, 197–8
    Awareness Model of Change 214–15
    Change agents 4, 62, 157, 174–80, 212, 221, 222, 244

Change programs 174–9
Change processes 23, 185–8, 191, 214, 216, 242
Change strategy 214–17
    Implicit criticism within any change 215
    Leading change 211–23 *passim*
    Promoting adaptive change 110, 190
    Vision Model of Change 214–16
    See also *Paradoxical Theory of Change*
Chaos 23, 51, 62, 125, 157
    Chaos Theory 5
Cheung-Judge, Mee-Yan xviii, 41, 263
Children xv, 7, 31, 80, 96–7, 127, 171, 174, 180
Closed systems 94
Closure 18, 21, 63, 157, 163, 201, 222, 253, 254, 261
Coaching xix, xx, 12, 19–20, 79, 90, 109–13, 119–22, 164, 179, 246
Cognition 200
Collective renewal 93, 95, 102
Collectivist values 167, 173, 175, 178–80
Collins, James 231
Collusion 16–17, 25
Comfort zone xiii, 82, 84, 85, 219
Communication 7, 88, 116–18, 171–3, 199, 202, 207–8
Competency 111, 154, 160, 162, 198, 209, 227, 230–2
Complexity xvii, xix, 51, 59, 62, 71, 77, 79, 83, 88–91, 101, 109, 124, 167, 199, 206, 210, 229
    Crisis of 188
Consciousness 229
Contact 52, 63, 88, 105, 148, 156, 170, 176, 180, 214, 221, 254
Context 229, 247
Continuous learning 8, 24, 59
Contracting 13, 24, 33, 66
Counter dependency 18–19

Covert processes 16
Cowie, Kate xix, 93, 263
Creative adaption 83, 88
Creative indifference (or 'void' or 'point of balance') 45
Creativity 31, 81, 112, 114, 120, 156, 200
Cultural assumptions 172, 174, 178
Culture 7, 87–8, 167–80 *passim*, 212, 228, 230, 233, 242–7
Curiosity ix, xiii, 81, 89, 136, 158, 160, 162, 219, 220, 222, 237
Cycle of Experience 3, 6, 44, 63, 66, 69, 88, 119, 156, 161, 164, 170, 201, 242, 245, 253, 254, 260, 261

Development, Socio-economic 167–9
Disruption 212
Dreams 120, 144, 179, 229, 254
Dream Work 254
Drucker, Peter F. 124, 209

Ecology 103, 258
Embodied values 113–14
Emotional intelligence 28, 110, 114, 120, 176, 180
Empathy 14, 33, 70, 97, 110, 120, 131, 176
Empty Chair (Experiment in Gestalt practice) 254, 255
Energy 14, 15, 17–20, 129, 141–51 *passim*, 156
Equilibrium 99
  Living equilibrium 78, 81
Exaggeration Exercise (Experiment in Gestalt practice) 254–5
Executive, Definition of 124
Executive coaching 12, 19, 20, 25, 123–40 *passim*
Executive's Gestalt 123–40 *passim*
Existentialism xv, 5, 255, 257
Experience xiv, 6, 59, 65–71 *passim*, 95–6, 110, 142, 154, 184, 212, 245
  Capacity for experiencing 70
  Concrete experience 59, 65–6, 255
  Personal experience, Power of 144–5

Experiential Learning Theory 59–71 *passim*, 87, 218, 255
Experimentation 18–20, 31, 43, 59, 64, 71, 119–20, 145, 147, 150, 163, 220, 254–5
  Active 59–60, 65, 66
Experiment in Gestalt practice 254–5, 258, 260

Failure 11, 24, 107, 110, 114, 119–20
Feedback 5, 52–3, 68, 87, 112–20 *passim*, 159, 164, 185–6, 198, 214–15
Fertile void 45, 255
Field Theory 14, 35, 42, 44, 49, 62, 168, 226, 228, 250, 254, 258, 261
Figure/ground xii–xiii, 45–6, 109, 119, 226–7, 237, 245
Fluidity 84, 88
Force field 14
Frank, Gudrun xx, 197, 263
Freud, Sigmund 17, 42–4, 46, 61, 168
Friedlander, Salomon 62, 254
FROGI (Four Roles of the Gestalt Intervener) 65–71
From, Isadore x, 4, 61, 257
Fuller, Stephen 11–17, 24
Funerals, Symbolic 21–2

General Electric 18
General Motors 11–13, 16, 24
Gestalt Institute of Cleveland viii, x, 4, 5, 8, 12, 21, 64, 144, 146, 153, 156, 168, 254
Gestalt Organization & Systems Development Program (OSD) 65, 168–9, 178, 241
Gestalt Organization and Systems Development 4–8, 62, 168, 241
Gestalt Prayer 170, 256
Gestalt Psychology or Gestaltism 14, 17, 27, 41–4, 60, 77, 93, 170, 250, 255, 256, 257
Gestalt Theory x–xiii, 4–5, 24, 45, 49, 60, 64, 109, 153, 167–9, 200, 211, 219, 225, 249
Gestalt Therapy xvii, 3–4, 8, 11–25

INDEX

passim, 32, 33, 41–5, 83, 93, 144, 170, 255, 256, 257
Globalization   xviii, 77, 90, 91, 107
Goodman, Paul   4, 43–5, 61, 144, 156, 168, 257
Goldstein, Kurt   42, 44, 257
Group-as-a-whole level analysis   17
Group dynamics   12, 17, 25, 168

Habit   34, 82, 154, 156, 157, 162, 257
Hanafin, Jonno   viii, xx, 48, 111, 146, 211, 263
Hefferline, Ralph   44, 144
Heifetz, Ronald   227, 231, 237
Heroes   87, 93, 98, 102
Hierarchy   87, 90, 155, 159, 177, 183, 189, 204, 243
Hirsch, Leonard   x
Hofstede, Geert   172, 178–80, 246–7
Holism   18, 30, 45, 51, 62, 77, 93–5, 230, 242, 249–52, 257
  Theory of   94
Homeostasis   193–4, 257
Hopkins, Walt   xix, 141, 264
Human development journey   95–7
Human moments   7
Human Resources (HR)   11–12, 14, 17, 202–3
Humanism   27, 30–6
Husserl, Edmund   42, 45

Identity   99–101, 111, 113, 167, 171, 179, 253
Impasse   27, 35–6
Inclusion   xvi, 45, 52, 71, 95, 97–8
Inertia   189–94
Influencing   60, 66, 68, 71, 146
Information Processing
  Systems   78–80
Inkoom, Daniel K.B.   xx, 241, 264
Integration   18, 22–4, 177
International Gestalt Organization and Leadership Development
  (iGOLD)   169, 178, 241, 256
Internet   6–7, 89
Intervention   xii, 4, 6, 18, 45, 47, 51–2, 62, 64, 67–8, 88, 104, 109, 119, 123, 139, 148, 161–4, 174, 257
Doing vs *being* interventions   111
Intuition   34, 36, 117–18, 128

Jones, Brenda B.   viii, ix, x, xvi, xx, 46, 47, 48, 111, 225, 264
Journey   ix, x, xiii, xvii, 24, 53, 93–7, 105, 141, 144, 216

Kegan, Robert   96, 99
Kepner, Elaine   viii, x, 19
Kierkegaard   42, 45
Koffka, Kurt   42, 60, 168
Kohler, Wolfgang   42, 60, 168
Kolb, David   59, 64, 69–71

Leadership   5, 87, 104, 106, 109–113, 120–21, 123–6, 140, 163, 168–9, 170–7, 212, 214, 216, 221, 241, 256
  African   173
  And Gestalt coaching   121
  And self-awareness   221
  Effective leadership   130
  Lewin's theories of   168
  Transformational   5
Leading vs managing   211
Learning cycles   64–5, 87
  Dual learning cycles   69
Learning processes   80, 88, 208–9
Leon, Janet   144
Letting go   15, 16, 21, 261
Levels of system   x, xiii, 3, 60, 78, 131, 204, 226, 228, 242–5, 248
Lewin, Kurt   xvii, 7, 14, 20, 42, 44, 52, 60–2, 88, 168, 226, 228, 250–1, 254, 256, 258, 261
Life space   52, 258
Loevinger, Jane   99, 101
Lohmeier, Jochen   169
Lukensmeyer, Carolyn J.   viii, ix, x, 264

Making the Rounds (Experiment in Gestalt Therapy)   258
Malone, Ollie, Jr.   xix, 123, 265
Marshak, Robert J.   249, 265
Maslow, Abraham   101, 105
McAfee, Andrew   228–9

271

Meaning making 34, 46, 93, 103, 156–7, 163, 227, 231, 235
Melnick, Joseph xix, 153, 155, 265
Mindfulness 27, 61, 62, 70, 81, 88, 90, 109, 115, 253
 Organizational mindfulness 88
Mission 23, 118, 121, 163, 179, 186–9, 231
Mjema, Nathaniel 169
Molini, Eugenio xix–xx, 183, 266
Multicultural contexts 7–9
Multiple realities xvi, 7, 45, 64, 71, 138, 150, 201, 206–7, 244, 258, 260

Nevis, Edwin C. vii, viii, ix, x, xviii, 3, 43, 47, 48, 63, 139, 150, 153, 266
 And use of self 46–7
Nevis, Sonia x, 146, 153
New York Institute for Gestalt Therapy 44
Nkum, John viii, xx, 169, 241, 266
Noticing 59, 66, 68, 70–1, 128, 136, 142, 147–50

Open mindedness 81, 84, 87, 88, 89, 90
Open systems 24, 94, 226
Openness 80, 81, 83–4, 89, 221
Optimism 116, 155–6, 258
Organism/Environment (O/E) xii, 4–5, 43–4, 49, 62, 78–9, 81, 103, 169–70, 211, 220, 226, 228, 248, 258
Organization and Systems Development (OSD) 4–8, 168, 241
Organization Development (OD) xiii, xvi, 11, 47, 61, 88, 167–8, 243–6, 249, 259
Organizational behavior xvii, 5, 11
Organizational culture(s) 85–8, 230, 243, 244, 246
Organizational purpose 104, 106

Paradoxical Theory of Change xix, 94, 109, 157, 214, 219, 259
Parent–child frameworks 180
Patterns 5, 14, 22, 63, 117, 137, 157, 162–4, 188, 234, 256, 260

Perceived Weirdness Index (PWI) 111, 118, 259
Perception 42, 77–9, 167–8, 258, 259, 260
 Theory of complex perception 41
Performance–Learning Dilemma 213
Perls, Fritz x, xvii, 3, 4, 8, 17, 27–8, 32, 35, 42–4, 60, 63, 94, 144, 156, 168, 210, 254, 256, 257, 258, 260
 And impasse 35
 Gestalt Prayer 170, 256
 vs Freud 17, 46
Perls, Laura x, 3, 4, 8, 32, 42–3, 61, 168, 257
Petrie, Nick 227
Phenomenology 42–5, 52, 226, 229, 259
Physical sensation 28–9, 142, 145, 147–9
Polster, Miriam 144–5, 147
Porras, Jerry 231
Power 17–18, 87, 90, 145–6, 155, 172, 177, 189, 243–5
Pragnanz xiii, 192, 202, 259
Praise and recognition 129
Presence xiii, 5, 28, 33, 36, 44–8, 60, 63, 110–12, 115, 119, 122, 129, 139, 146, 155, 159–60, 176, 259
 Holistic 60, 69–70
 Relational 46, 111
Present, The 16, 20, 28, 35, 109, 154, 160, 162, 190, 192, 229, 259
Process, Emphasis on 6, 36, 62, 66, 162, 190, 212, 214, 250
Process consultation 12, 68
Process tools 119–21
Professionalisation (of Gestalt) 27, 30, 32–6, 44
Projection 28–9, 33, 112, 119, 215, 254, 260
Psychic immune system 80, 81, 85, 90
Psychodynamic theory 17, 261

Rainey, Mary Ann viii, ix, x, xvi, xviii, 3, 46–8, 59, 111, 146, 266
Ramo, Joshua Cooper 225
Recruitment 169, 203

INDEX

Reich, Wilhelm 43, 45
Relationships 130
Relaxation 81, 84–5, 142, 158, 162
Requisite variety 112
Resilience 88, 91, 155–6, 194, 225
Resistance 4, 15, 34, 61, 64, 109–10, 144, 148–50, 157–8, 186, 189–91, 194, 197, 219–20, 242–4, 259
    As immune system 219
    Eliminating use of the word 7
    Seven learnings on resistance 149
    Working with 3, 64, 149
Restructuring 217
Reversal Technique (Experiment in Gestalt Therapy) 260
Rewards 217
Roettgers, Eva x, xix, 77, 267
Role modelling 216–17

"Safe emergency" 64, 145, 147, 220
Sapolsky, Robert 174, 180
Schein, Edgar 230
Scientific methods 31, 41–2, 44
Seeing and being seen 148
Seeing oneself 131
Self, The 42, 45–51, 93, 96–7, 99–102, 113
    As resource 46
    Search for 93, 102
    Also see Use of self
Self, Other and Situation (SOS) 49–51
Self-actualisation 28, 31, 34, 36, 49, 101, 105, 258
Self-awareness 47, 51, 52, 110, 112–14, 120–1, 176, 221, 257, 260
Self-care 130
Self-interest 94, 103, 172
Self-organizing systems 5
Self-reflection 50, 115, 118, 198
Sensation 47, 52, 63, 65, 81, 113, 119, 141, 142, 156, 170, 245, 254, 260
Senses, The five human 135, 142
Siminovitch, Dorothy E. xix, 267
Small talk 161
Social structure 17
Solms, Mark 170
Spirituality 27–30, 95, 98–102, 221, 229

Stakeholder engagement 66, 88, 104, 169, 187, 194, 205, 212, 228
Strategy 212
Streams of Development 98–9
Stress 70, 82–5, 120, 175, 205, 215
Stress zone 82
"Success" 12, 129
Survival zone 83
System, Levels of 4, 67, 105, 119, 200, 204, 206, 228
Systemic approach 184, 191, 193, 204, 227, 234, 247
Systems Theory xiii, xix, 5, 44, 61, 94, 103, 226, 256, 260

T Groups 12, 64, 148, 259
Team building 12
Tension xix–xx, 78–9, 90, 142, 167, 173, 178, 185, 188, 211, 225, 243
Theme 62, 68, 70–1, 78, 137, 175, 214, 220, 245, 250, 260
Threat 118, 155, 186, 219
Top Dog/Under Dog (Experiment in Gestalt Therapy) 260
Theorizing
    Grand Theorizing 60, 66–8, 71
Tragedy of the commons 94
Transcendence 33, 95, 98
Transference 28, 29, 46
Transformational leadership 5
Trust 64, 113, 158–9, 189, 222
    And learning 158

Ubuntu 171
Unit of work 3, 63, 66, 69, 119, 199, 201, 205, 209, 212–13, 261
Unfinished business 18, 20–2, 83, 115, 222
Unresolved issues 13, 20–1
Use of group 141, 146–7, 150
Use of self xiii, xvi, 4, 41, 46–8, 50, 53, 61, 63, 109, 111–12, 119–22, 144, 146–8, 150, 176, 221, 259

Vision statements 214, 216
Voice 116–17
Von Ehrenfels, Christian 41, 60

Wertheimer, Max   42, 168, 259
Whole Thinking Approach   202–4, 208–9
Wholeness   xiii, 33, 46, 95, 173, 177, 202
Withdrawal   63, 156, 254, 261
World centrism   96–7, 101–7

Wundt, Wilhelm   41
Wyley, Chantelle   viii, xix, 167, 267

Zeigarnik, Bluma   20, 168, 261
Zeigarnik Effect   20, 261
Zen   27–8, 33, 35
Zinker, Joseph   21, 27–8, 32

www.ingramcontent.com/pod-product-compliance
Lightning Source LLC
Chambersburg PA
CBHW071223080526
44587CB00013BA/1474